Advances in
Ultrasound Techniques
and Instrumentation

CLINICS IN DIAGNOSTIC ULTRASOUND VOLUME 28

Volumes Already Published

Advances in Ultrasound Techniques and Instrumentation

Edited by

Peter N. T. Wells, Ph.D., D.Sc., F. Eng.

Chief Physicist
Department of Medical Physics
Bristol General Hospital
United Bristol Healthcare Trust
Honorary Professor
Department of Medical Physics
University of Bristol Faculty of Medicine
Bristol, England

Churchill Livingstone
New York, Edinburgh, London, Madrid, Melbourne, Tokyo

Library of Congress Cataloging-in-Publication Data
Advances in ultrasound techniques and instrumentation / edited by
    Peter N.T. Wells.
        p. cm. — (Clinics in diagnostic ultrasound ; v. 28)
    Includes bibliographical references and index.
    ISBN 0-443-08853-5
    1. Diagnosis, Ultrasonic. I. Wells, P. N. T. (Peter Neil Temple)
  II. Series.
    [DNLM: 1. Ultrasonography—instrumentation. 2. Ultrasonography—
  methods. W1 CL831BC v.28 1993 / WB 289 A244 1993]
  RC78.7U4A38 1993
  616.07'54—dc20
  DNLM/DLC
  for Library of Congress   92-48481
                                                    CIP

Distributed in the United Kingdom by Churchill Livingstone, Robert Stevenson House,
1–3 Baxter's Place, Leith Walk, Edinburgh EH1 3AF, and by associated companies, branches, and representatives throughout the world.

Accurate indications, adverse reactions, and dosage schedules for drugs are provided in this
book, but it is possible that they may change. The reader is urged to review the package
information data of the manufacturers of the medications mentioned.

The Publishers have made every effort to trace the copyright holders for borrowed material
If they have inadvertently overlooked any, they will be pleased to make the necessary
arrangements at the first opportunity.

Acquisitions Editor: *Nancy Mullins*
Copy Editor: *Paul Bernstein*
Production Designer: *Patricia McFadden*
Production Supervisor: *Jeanine Furino*

Printed in the United States of America

First published in 1993   7 6 5 4 3 2 1

Contributors

Jeffrey C. Bamber, Ph.D.

Lecturer, Faculty of Biophysics, University of London, London, England; Leader, Investigative Ultrasound Team, Joint Department of Physics, Institute of Cancer Research and Royal Marsden Hospital, Sutton, Surrey, England

Nicolaas Bom, Ph.D.

Professor, Division of Medical Technology, Thoraxcentre, Department of Cardiology, Erasmus University Rotterdam; Interuniversity Cardiology Institute of the Netherlands, Rotterdam, the Netherlands

Pieter D. Brommersma, M.Sc.

Research Fellow, Thoraxcentre, Department of Cardiology, Erasmus University Rotterdam, Rotterdam, the Netherlands

David H. Evans, Ph.D.

Professor, Department of Medical Physics, School of Medicine, University of Leicester; Head of Service, Department of Medical Physics, Leicester Royal Infirmary, Leicester, England

Barry B. Goldberg, M.D.

Professor, Department of Radiology, Jefferson Medical College of Thomas Jefferson University; Director, Division of Diagnostic Ultrasound, Department of Radiology, Thomas Jefferson University Hospital, Philadelphia, Pennsylvania

Timothy J. Hall, Ph.D.

Assistant Professor, Department of Diagnostic Radiology, University of Kansas Medical Center School of Medicine, Kansas City, Kansas

Rachel A. Harris, M.Sc.

Senior Physicist, Vascular Studies Unit, Royal United Hospital, Combe Park, Bath, England

Christy K. Holland, Ph.D.

Associate Research Scientist, Ultrasound Section, Department of Diagnostic Imaging, Yale University School of Medicine, New Haven, Connecticut

H. K. Huang, D.Sc., F.R.C.R. (Hon.)

Professor and Vice Chairman and Director, Laboratory for Radiologic Informatics, Department of Radiology, University of California, San Francisco, School of Medicine, San Francisco, California

Michael F. Insana, Ph.D.

Assistant Professor, Department of Diagnostic Radiology, University of Kansas City Medical Center School of Medicine, Kansas City, Kansas

Charles T. Lancée, M.Sc., Ph.D.

Research Associate, Thoraxcentre, Department of Cardiology, Erasmus University Rotterdam, Rotterdam, the Netherlands

Leonardo Masotti, Ph.D.

Professor and Director, Department of Electronic Engineering, University of Florence; Head, Ultrasound and Non-Destructive Testing Laboratory, Florence, Italy

W. Norman McDicken, Ph.D.

Professor, Department of Medical Physics and Medical Engineering, University of Edinburgh, Edinburgh, Scotland

Riccardo Pini, M.D.

Assistant Professor, Institute of Gerontology and Geriatrics, University of Florence, Florence, Italy; Adjunct Assistant Professor, Department of Cardiology, Cornell University Medical College, New York, New York

Peter F. Sharp, B.Sc, Ph.D., C.Phys., F.Inst.P., F.I.P.S.M.

Professor, Department of Bio-Medical Physics and Bio-Engineering, University of Aberdeen; Consultant Medical Physicist, Department of Bio-Medical Physics and Bio-Engineering, Aberdeen Royal Hospitals NHS Trust, Foresterhill, Aberdeen, Scotland

Thomas L. Szabo, Ph.D.

Senior Research Scientist, Imaging Systems Division, Hewlett Packard, Andover, Massachusetts

Kenneth J. W. Taylor, M.D., Ph.D., F.A.C.P.

Professor, Department of Diagnostic Imaging, Yale University School of Medicine; Director, Vascular Laboratory, Yale-New Haven Hospital, New Haven, Connecticut

Peter N. T. Wells, Ph.D., D.Sc., F.Eng.

Chief Physicist, Department of Medical Physics, Bristol General Hospital, United Bristol Healthcare Trust; Honorary Professor, Department of Medical Physics, University of Bristol Faculty of Medicine, Bristol, England

Marvin C. Ziskin, M.D., B.S.Bm.

Professor, Department of Diagnostic Imaging, Director, Center for Biomedical Physics, Temple University School of Medicine, Philadelphia, Pennsylvania

Preface

It is a rare event for a book in the *Clinics in Diagnostic Ultrasound* series to be devoted solely to physics and instrumentation. It has happened only once before, when I had the pleasure of being joined by Marvin Ziskin as co-editor of *New Techniques and Instrumentation in Ultrasonography*, which was published in 1980. *Advances in Ultrasound Techniques and Instrumentation* contains, like its predecessor, chapters that have been chosen to present a multifaceted view of the most exciting contemporary developments.

Nowadays the technology of medical imaging is at the forefront of the application of advanced physics and engineering. The authors of the chapters that make up this book have been mindful of the fact that it will be read mainly by radiologists and other physicians actively interested in diagnostic ultrasound. They have not shied away, however, from approaching the relevant physics and mathematics head-on. The result is that they have been extremely successful in writing reviews of their specialty subjects that can confidently be expected to be valuable not only as comprehensive reports but also as sources of reference leading to detailed studies of the related literature.

It is a pleasure for me to record my gratitude to all my friends who so graciously responded to my invitation to contribute to this volume. My task as editor was made easier by their willingness to comply with the discipline imposed by the publishers, to whom I am also grateful for their efficiency and encouragement.

Peter N. T. Wells, Ph.D., D.Sc., F.Eng.

Contents

Advances in
Ultrasound Techniques
and Instrumentation

Color Plates

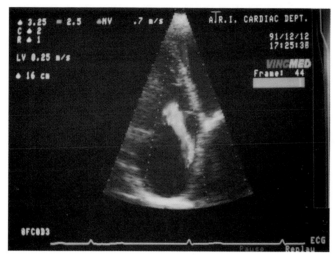

Plate 1-1

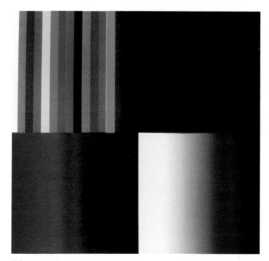

Plate 1-2

Plate 1-1 Doppler of cardiac chambers; red and blue indicate flow toward and away from the probe, respectively. Yellow indicates a disturbance to flow, in this case resulting from valvular regurgitation.

Plate 1-2 Various color scales used to represent image intensity. **Upper left,** contrasting colors; **bottom left,** uniform chromaticity; **bottom right,** hot-body scale.

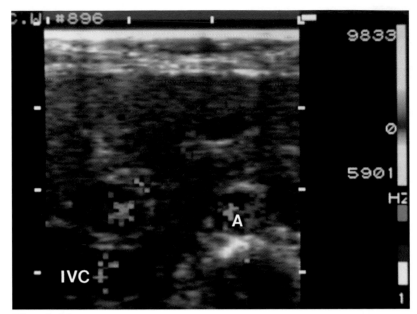

Plate 3–1A

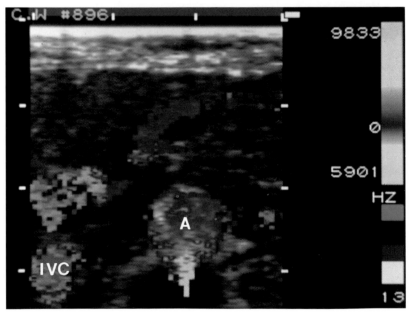

Plate 3–1B

Plate 3–1 Differences in color Doppler signals of intrahepatic arteries. **(A)** Aorta (A) and inferior vena cava (IVC) just before and **(B)** after the peripheral intravenous injection of air-filled albumin (Albunex).

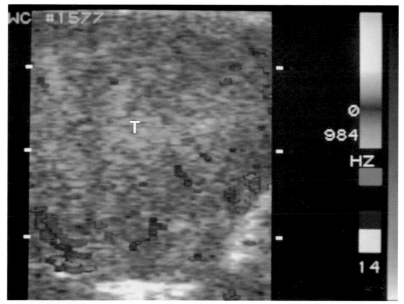

Plate 3-2A

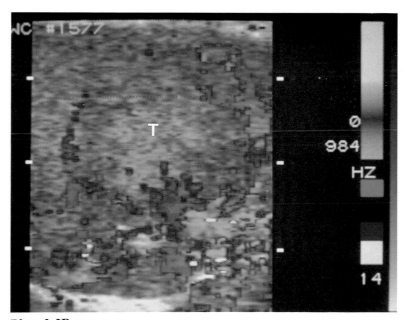

Plate 3-2B

Plate 3-2 Differences in color Doppler signals **(A)** just before and **(B)** after peripheral intravenous injection of air-filled albumin (Albunex). Color Doppler signal enhancement is seen around the periphery of the woodchuck hepatocellular tumor (T). At autopsy, the central area of the tumor was found to be undergoing necrosis, accounting for the lack of flow in this region. (From Goldberg B, Hilpert P, Burns P et al: Hepatic tumors: signal enhancement of Doppler US after intravenous injection of a contrast agent. Radiology 177:713, 1990, with permission.)

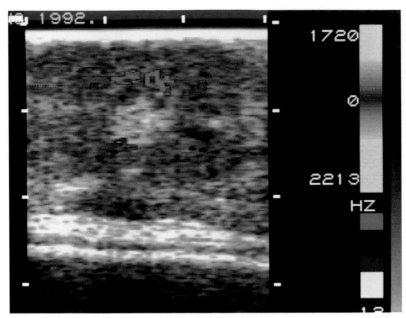

Plate 3-3A

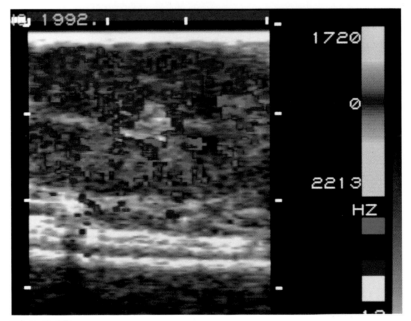

Plate 3-3B

Plate 3-3 **(A)** Before and **(B)** after peripheral intravenous injection of 1.0 ml SHU 508 (Levovist), demonstrating color Doppler signal enhancement in small vessels of a dog kidney.

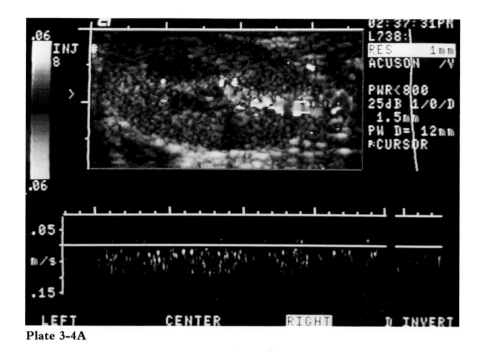

Plate 3-4A

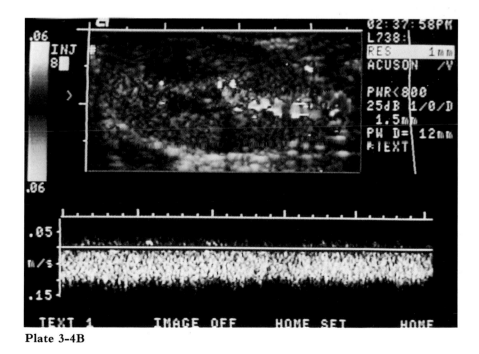

Plate 3-4B

Plate 3-4 Doppler spectrum of renal vein in a woodchuck shows longevity of Doppler signal enhancement after peripheral intravenous injection of 1.0 ml SHU 508 (Levovist). **(A)** Before injection. **(B)** Twenty seconds after injection. (*Figure continues.*)

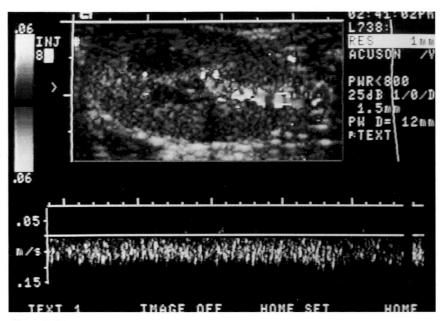

Plate 3-4C

Plate 3-4 (*Continued*). **(C)** Two hundred seconds after injection.

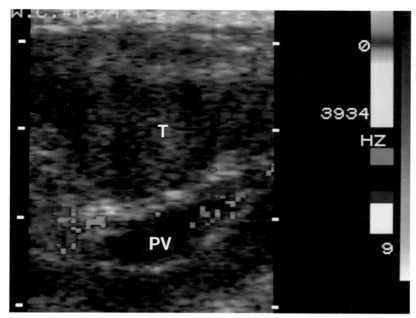

Plate 3-5A

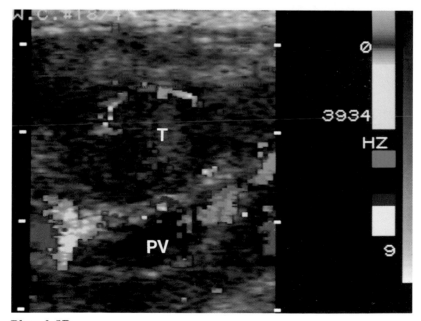

Plate 3-5B

Plate 3-5 Color Doppler signal enhancement is seen within a woodchuck hepatocellular tumor (T). **(A)** Before and **(B)** after peripheral intravenous injection of 1.0 ml SHU 508 (Levovist). Note the appearance of tumor vessels within the poorly-defined solid mass. PV, portal vein.

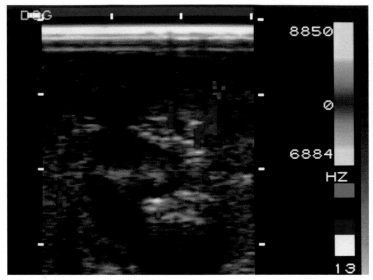

Plate 3-6A

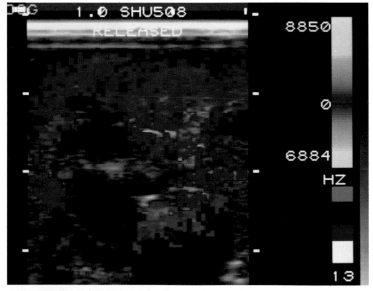

Plate 3-6B

Plate 3-6 Color Doppler signal enhancement can be seen in a dog kidney following peripheral intravenous injection of 1.0 ml SHU 508 (Levovist). **(A)** Before injection. **(B)** After injection. (*Figure continues.*)

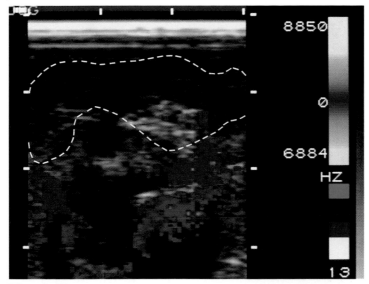

Plate 3-6C

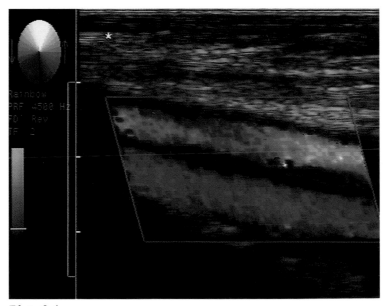

Plate 8-1

Plate 3-6 *(Continued)*. **(C)** After injection with ligation of a segmental renal artery. Note lack of flow in ischemic region (dotted area).

Plate 8-1 Color-flow image of a superficial femoral artery overlying a superficial femoral vein, produced with a linear array transducer (pulse-echo frequency, 5 MHz; Doppler imaging frequency, 4 MHz). Note that the "color box" is steered at an angle of 15 degrees relative to the gray-scale image.

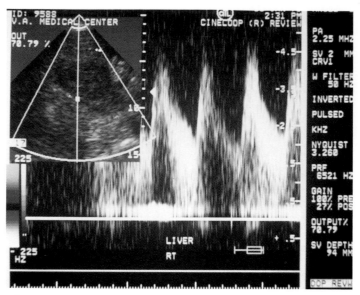

Plate 10-1

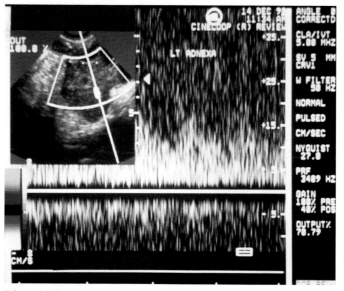

Plate 10-2

Plate 10-1 Color and pulse Doppler examination of focal liver lesion. Neovascularity is seen at edge of mass. Pulse Doppler shows systolic velocity of 4.5 kHz (3-MHz carrier frequency) and RI of 0.44. Such high Doppler shifts are characteristic of hepatomas.

Plate 10-2 Color and pulse Doppler examination of ovary in a postmenopausal woman. Peak systolic velocities are 18 cm/s; the RI is 0.44. Such flow is highly abnormal in a woman of this age and is consistent with ovarian cancer.

1

Display and Perception of Ultrasound Images

Peter F. Sharp

The clinical value of ultrasound is firmly recognized, ranking alongside radiography, nuclear medicine, and magnetic resonance imaging (MRI) as a well-established routine diagnostic imaging procedure. Yet in some respects it has developed in a unique way. The sine qua non for medical imaging systems is that they should provide volumetric data in a digital format. Although the image of a slice of data is provided, few attempts have been made in ultrasound to provide three-dimensional volumetric data. Also, although ultrasound data are, at one stage, stored in a digital form, relatively little advantage is taken of the potential for improving image quality by digital data processing and display; even conventional image processing facilities can be provided only as add-on, nonstandard equipment.

Thus, at first sight, the display and presentation of ultrasound images appears to be lacking in sophistication. However, the ability to produce real-time images with few constraints on imaging time is a real advantage not found with other medical imaging modalities. The interrogative nature of this process places greater demands on the person performing the imaging; it is not simply a matter of taking a picture to be viewed at a later date by a trained radiologist. Also any form of image processing that cannot be implemented in near real-time will slow down imaging significantly and will take from ultrasound one of its principal strengths.

Few attempts have been made to study the process of image presentation in ultrasound, probably because its nature makes it less amenable to a rigorous scientific study using images of relatively simple phantoms lacking anatomic realism. Ultrasound imaging also suffers from one other complication: the variation of spatial resolution in both the axial and transaxial directions means that it cannot be treated simply as a linear and spatially invariant imaging system. Thus the approaches adopted with other modalities, such as the use of the transfer function to describe spatial performance, cannot be readily used.

However, there are also many similarities between the problems encountered over data presentation and display in ultrasound and with other imaging modalities. First, all systems rely on the human observer, and so consideration must be given to matching display characteristics to those of the visual system. Second, at its simplest, the problem of signal detection is one of discriminating between image detail and noise. Speckle "noise," combined with electronic noise, is ultimately the limiting process for low-contrast signal detection.

DISPLAY SYSTEMS IN ULTRASOUND

The display of the standard ultrasound B-scan image poses several problems. The acquired data require significant modification before they are displayed in order to deal with the wide dynamic range of reflected signals, typically 120 dB, and there must be compensation for the attenuation experienced by signals reflected from structures deep in the body.

Typically, displays that use a gray scale to represent signal intensity can deal with a signal dynamic range of 35 to 40 dB; therefore considerable data compression is required. This can be carried out either as part of the receiver amplifier stage or when the acquired data are mapped onto the display. The latter case, postacquisition processing, has the obvious advantage of permitting the operator to judge whether the image contains all the relevant diagnostic information. However, although quite complex forms of data compression can be carried out, there is little guidance as to the best way to achieve optimum data display.

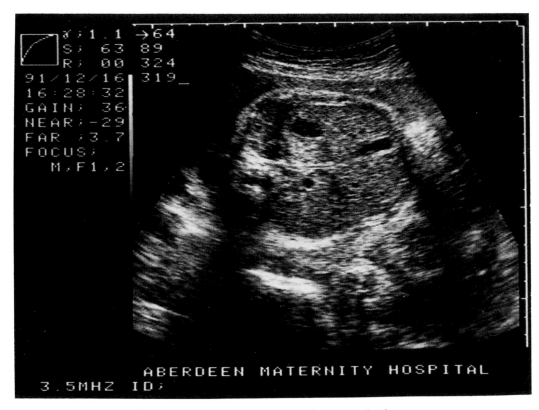

Fig. 1-1 B-scan image showing abdomen of a fetus.

The time-gain compensation, or swept gain control, alters the echo strength to a degree that depends on the depth from which it has been reflected. This can be performed automatically, in which case the processing is such that, on average, signal strength is independent of the depth from which the echo has been returned. Whereas manual controls allow the operator to achieve what is the supposedly best form of correction, this carries the obvious disadvantage that inappropriate corrections might result.

Both data compression and adjustment by the swept gain control change image contrast. In addition, the overall gain of the receiver amplifier can be varied, changing the absolute image brightness, and display monitor controls allow adjustment of contrast and brightness.

Finally, but certainly not of the least significance, one must consider the composition of the image itself. Because features result from reflections at interfaces, there is an accentuation of the edges of structures. Noise is predominantly coherent speckle, its form depending on the characteristics of the scanner as well as the structure of the organs being imaged. At low intensities, electronic noise predominates.

Although gray-scale coding of signal intensity is widely used (Fig. 1-1), color-coded flow data are superimposed on the gray-scale image in Doppler (Plate 1-1). There is, thus, significant potential for operator interaction, both in the way in which the data are displayed and in the selection of which data are acquired. Before considering the factors influencing data display, we first consider the behavior of the human visual system.

THE HUMAN OBSERVER

At present, the ultrasound pulse-echo is interrogated by the human observer. How effectively the image data are interpreted depends on the combination of the basic "performance" of the visual system and the ability of the observer to understand the complex data in the image. The two are not independent, as obviously interpretation depends on the quality of the information received (i.e., how well the visual system performs).

For ultrasound images, we are interested in four aspects of the visual system performance: its ability to detect small changes in gray level, its temporal response, its spatial response, and the perception of color. Also crucial to image interpretation is the need for the observer to make a decision; this is not a simple process and is considered separately in a later section.

Visual System

The anatomy of the eye is illustrated in Figure 1-2A. The cornea, aqueous, lens, and vitreous are known as the ocular refractive media. The effective power of the eye is approximately 60 diopters (i.e., it has a focal length of about 1.6 cm), with the cornea being the strongest refractive element, having an effective power of about 45 diopters, whereas the lens has a power of about 15 diopters in its unaccommodated state.

Like any optical system, the eye suffers from various aberrations, which have been compensated for in several ways. The curvature of the cornea is steepest in its center and flattens near the periphery, helping to reduce spherical aberration and oblique astigmatism. The iris acts as a stop, limiting the entry of peripheral rays into the eye. The optimum pupil size is 2.0 to 2.5 mm; above this value, image quality is degraded by spherical aberration, whereas below it, quality is affected by diffraction.

The retina itself (Fig. 1-2B) also plays a part in correcting image data. The retinal cones are more sensitive to light striking them axially than obliquely; this is the so-called Stiles-Crawford effect,[2] and it reduces spher-

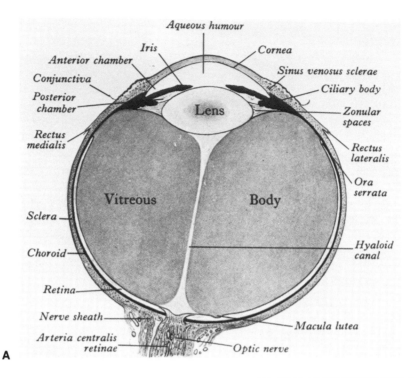

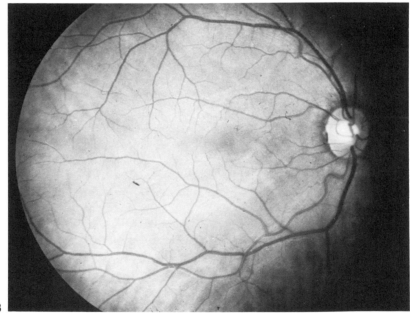

Fig. 1-2 (A) Horizontal section through a human eyeball. **(B)** Normal right retina. (Fig. A from Warwick and Williams,[1] with permission.)

ical aberration. The periphery of the retina has relatively poor resolution and thus minimizes the effect of astigmatic images. Finally, the curvature of the retina compensates for the curvature of field produced by the optical system.

Light falling on the retina is absorbed by visual pigments contained in the photoreceptors, of which there are two types, the rods and cones, so called because of their shapes. There are approximately 120 million rods in the retina, all situated outside the fovea, and 6 million cones, mostly in the fovea and parafoveal regions. Although the rods have a spectral sensitivity peak at 500 nm, the cones contain one of three pigments, with peaks at 450 nm (blue cones), 525 nm (green cones), and 555 nm (red cones).

In addition to these photoreceptors, the retina contains four other groups of cells: bipolar, ganglion, horizontal, and amacrine cells. Ganglion cells have specific receptive fields in which a stimulus evokes a train of neural impulses. There is a variety of such fields. In the on-center, off-surround type, the onset of illumination of the center of the receptive field causes the neural pulse rate to increase, although it is only when illumination of the surround is switched off that a response is produced. Other cells have off-center, on-surround fields in which the roles of center and surround are reversed. Another type of ganglion cell responds to a stimulus moving within its receptive field, the response being directionally selective. This signal processing is brought about by the other cells. For example, the concentric receptive field is the result of lateral inhibition of bipolar cell output by the horizontal cells, whereas amacrine cells are associated with the temporal responses shown by some ganglion cells.

The axons of the ganglion cells form the optic nerve. At the optic chiasm, the optic nerves from the two eyes meet, and the axons subserving the nasal half of the retina cross into the contralateral optic tract. It is this cross-over that produces the visual field topography. The optic nerve axons pass through the optic tracts to synapse in the lateral geniculate nucleus (LGN), a subnucleus of the thalamus.

The LGN consists of six cytoarchitectural layers; the four dorsal layers consist of small (parvo) cells and the two ventral layers are large-cell (magnocellular) layers. Each eye projects to three layers in an alternating fashion. These two types of cells receive inputs from two intermixed but anatomically distinct types of retinal ganglion cells. These two divisions of the visual pathway are referred to as the *magno* and *parvo*.[3]

The magno and parvo systems have many differences in their behavior; the magno cell response is achromatic, has a much higher contrast sensitivity, responds more quickly, but has a larger receptive field. However, significantly they have some common characteristics. The receptive fields are circularly symmetric, and most show either the on-center off-surround or off-center on-surround characteristics mentioned earlier. This emphasizes the important role played by edges and other discontinuities in illumination in providing perceptual information.

From the LGN, the visual pathway consists of the optic radiations through the parietal and temporal lobes, terminating in the primary visual cortex in the occipital lobe. These divisions then appear to continue into the higher visual area: a full discussion of their anatomy and physiology is found elsewhere.[3]

Color Vision

As has been mentioned, there are three types of cones with visual pigments having sensitivity peaks at either 450 nm (blue cones), 525 nm (green cones), or 555 nm (red cones) but having a broad band response. The so-called trichromatic component theory of color vision is based on the observation that any color can be matched by a mixture of three primary colors (i.e., red, green, and blue).[4] However, to achieve this match it may be necessary to subtract one color from the others and not simply to add colors. Information on hue is provided by the ratio of the outputs from the red, green, and blue receptors, whereas saturation and brightness is determined by the sum of the outputs.

However, although the trichromatic theory explains color matching, it does not address the problem of how a color looks to an observer. For example, a color never appears both reddish and greenish, although it may look both greenish and bluish. The opponent theory of color vision[5] is based on the presence of three pairs of detectors acting in opposition: two of these deal with color, one corresponding to red and green and the other to yellow (i.e., red plus green) and blue. The third is a black–white opponent system, primarily for brightness and saturation. The red–green detector signals the presence of either red or green wavelengths but gives no indication of the yellow or blue ones. If the red input predominates, the output of the red–green system is positive (i.e., above baseline levels), whereas if green is greater, the output is negative. There is support for the presence of a mechanism at the level of the LGN.

At present, the most likely model for color vision is one containing elements of both component and opponent theories; the red, green, and blue receptor signals are handled separately up to the level of the LGN, where they then are combined through the lateral inhibitory networks.[6] Opponent color coding then is assumed to continue to the cortex.

A third channel is required to signal luminance. The red and green, but probably not the blue, signals are added. This channel is also opponent-coded and signals not the absolute luminance but how the local value compares with the luminance across the rest of the image. Comparisons are made across space rather than color. This explains color constancy, where our perception of color depends largely on the object's spectral reflectance characteristics rather than the spectral composition of the illuminating light.[7]

Physical Performance of the Visual System

SPATIAL RESPONSE

The ability of an imaging system to record spatial information can be expressed in terms of the optical transfer function.[8] However, this assumes that linear systems theory can be applied, but unfortunately this is not valid for the visual system. Although its response is reasonably homogeneous near the optic axis, in other parts of the visual field it is anisotropic with the response to a test pattern being dependent on its orientation.[9] The response of the eye to spatial detail is also dependent on the contrast of the input pattern.

However, if measurements are confined to one area of the retina and made at low contrast, a curve such as that shown in Figure 1-3A results. This shows the relative sensitivity of response of the visual system to a

---

Fig. 1-3 (A) Contrast sensitivity curve for the human eye. The visual system is most sensitive to spatial frequencies of a few cycles per degree. To see spatial information of a fraction of a cycle per degree or several tens of cycles, image contrast has to increase by one or two orders of magnitude. **(B)** Curves showing how sensitivity of the visual system varies with the temporal frequency with which a stimulus is presented. At high frequencies, the ability to perceive flicker is independent of average brightness. (Fig. A from Campbell and Maffei,[10] with permission. Fig. B from Kelly,[14] with permission.)

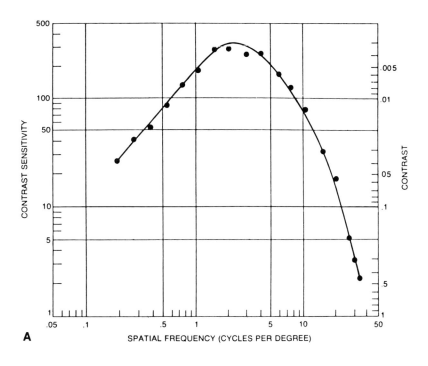

A

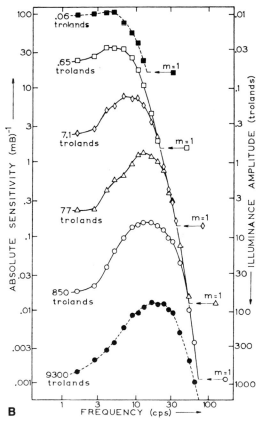

B

sine-wave pattern. The precise shape of the curve and its cut-off frequency depend on how measurements are made and the absolute brightness levels used.

The visual system is most sensitive to spatial frequencies of about 15 cycles per degree and sensitivity falls off rapidly at both higher and lower frequencies, the cut-off frequency being about 60 cycles per degree. This decrease is not dependent on the properties of the cornea and lens[11] but is probably a function of the size of the receptors. At high spatial frequencies, the summation of outputs from rods degrades resolution, as also does scatter of light. The latter is, however, reduced by the Stiles-Crawford effect. The low frequency response is a result of the process of lateral inhibition, which effectively filters out low spatial frequencies.

Although we may not be aware of this limitation of the visual system in reproducing spatial information in a scene, it can lead to some unusual effects in images, the most notable being the Mach band phenomenon.[12] More relevant to ultrasound imaging is that it explains why, in some circumstances, the display raster pattern may be visually intrusive. Although this problem has not been addressed in ultrasound, Pitt et al.[13] demonstrated how the appearance of digitized nuclear medicine images can be improved by varying the image spatial frequency content by image minification so that those frequencies associated with the edges of individual picture elements correspond to the tails of the contrast sensitivity function and therefore are "seen" only poorly.

TEMPORAL RESPONSE

The temporal response of the visual system—how rapidly it can react to changes in illumination—is measured in terms of the critical flicker frequency or critical fusion frequency.[14] The temporal equivalent to Figure 1-3A is shown in Figure 1-3B, spatial frequency being replaced by temporal frequency. As can be seen, the maximum flicker rate detectable by the eye is about 60 Hz. This effect is used in the ciné presentation of images.

DYNAMIC RANGE

The eye is capable of performing over a dynamic range of about 10^{13}. For a dynamic range of about 10^4, its performance remains constant, but over the remainder it gradually deteriorates. This performance is achieved by a combination of four mechanisms. First, the rods and cones have different sensitivities to light; vision at low light levels primarily uses the rods with consequent loss of acuity. Second, there is summation of many rods to a single ganglion cell, which improves performance at low light levels. Third, there is a chemical gain control (dark adaptation), but this changes relatively slowly. Finally, the lens aperture, the iris, can vary rapidly, giving a gain control of a factor of about 64.

Perception

The previous discussion has concentrated on the anatomy and physiology of the eye and its performance as an optical instrument. However, this is only the first step so far as the display and interpretation of information is concerned. Perception can be considered as having five developmental stages[15]:

1. The stage of light detection
2. Realization that an unspecified object is present in the visual field; the stage of the generic object
3. Appreciation that there is a contoured figure in some specific part of the visual field; the stage of the differentiated object
4. Visualization of an object with a specific form or shape and having a detailed outline; the stage of the specific object
5. Previous experience influences the interpretation of the object; the stage of manipulation

In terms of the physiology of the visual system, the parvo cellular system seems to be selective for form and color, whereas depth and movement information are linked to the magno system.

Basic to all these processes of perception, with perhaps the exception of the first stage, is the ability to differentiate between the relevant information in the image and that which is irrelevant to the particular task that is being carried out. This leads to the problems of decision making.

DECISION MAKING

The potential for the viewer to use the information from a display is fundamentally determined by the performance of the visual system as described in the previous section. However, the actual performance achieved also depends on the ability of the observer to use this information in making a decision.

Consider the simple problem of determining the performance of a display system in terms of the minimum contrast needed to detect the presence of a signal. The information received by the visual system can be regarded as constituting a visual stimulus of a particular strength, measured on some arbitrary scale. At one time it was assumed that the observer adopted some internal sensory threshold; for correct completion of the task, in this case for the signal to be seen, the visual stimulus must exceed this fixed threshold value. However, it was appreciated that the input received from the signal was variable; presenting stimuli of the same average intensity did not always produce the same visual effect. As the average signal intensity increased, the probability of the observer giving the correct answer also increased. This situation is represented diagrammatically in Figure 1-4. Thus, for a particular task, it was possible to measure the performance of the display in terms of the contrast needed for

the signal to be detected. Effectively one was measuring performance in terms of the position of the visual threshold.

This viewpoint was challenged by Tanner and Swets,[16] who demonstrated that the visual threshold was not fixed but could be *consciously* varied by the observer. In particular, as the degree of confidence required of the observer in making a decision was increased, the visual threshold also increased (i.e., the intensity needed for the signal to be seen increased). The implication of this was that display performance could not be measured precisely in terms of the signal contrast required for detection. Instead, an approach was needed that would separate the effect of choice of the observer's decision criterion from that of the stimulus produced by the displayed signal.

Signal Detection Theory

The basic premise of this approach is that the observer can alter the threshold depending on the degree of confidence that he or she has in the decision. To return to the visual stimulus concept, we now must represent the (variable) decision-making process as involving a series of visual thresholds. Thus, for a given displayed signal, the measured true-positive response rate varies depending on the observer's confidence in the decision. Differences in display performance might well be caused by changes in the decision criterion rather than the effectiveness with which the data are presented, so it may appear that there is no way of discriminating between the effect produced by the decision process and the visual stimulus produced by the displayed signal.

Another way of looking at the quality of the displayed image is in terms of its ability to allow the observer to differentiate between an image containing the signal and one that has no signal in it. At this point it is not necessary to be specific as to what constitutes a

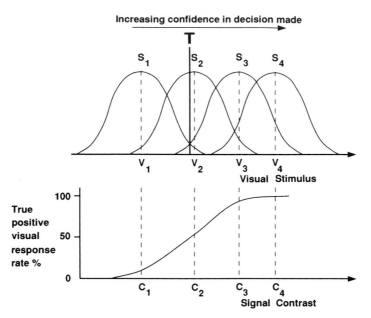

Fig. 1-4 Image whose mean signal strength is S_1 (corresponding to an image contrast of C_1) produces a visual impression (or stimulus) on the observer of mean value V_1. Variability in the appearance of the image is indicated by Gaussian probability density curves associated with each signal. Observer is assumed to adopt some threshold value, T, such that if visual stimulus exceeds it, the signal is seen. Position of T depends on the confidence of the observer in his or her decision. As mean signal strength increases, so does probability that the signal will be seen (i.e., true-positive visual response). Experimentally one obtains a plot of signal contrast against visual response rate and from this chooses, fairly arbitrarily, contrast at which the signal can be said to be seen. Position of this **S**-shaped curve depends on threshold, observer's decision criterion, and visual impression produced by the displayed signal.

signal (e.g., it may be the presence of a simple abnormal area in an image or as complex as a group of clinical features that allows us to state that the image represents a cirrhotic rather than normal liver). In the terminology of signal detection theory, we measure the performance of a display by its ability to permit the observer to differentiate between signals and noise; noise refers to an image that does not contain the signal and not necessarily to the random fluctuations in the ultrasound signal.

The visual stimulus produced by the noise also can be represented by a probability distribution (Fig. 1-5A). As the threshold varies, the proportion of noise distribution and the proportion of signal distribution exceeding the threshold change. The former produces the false-positive response rate and the latter produces the true-positive rate. By plotting true-positive rate against false-positive rate, we generate a curve known as the receiver operating characteristic (ROC) curve.

Given a particular task, the better of two displays is the one whose representation of the data produces the more effective differentiation between signal and noise distributions. As these distributions move apart, the corresponding ROC curves shift toward the top left-hand corner of the graph (Fig. 1-5B).

A description of how to measure these curves experimentally has been given by Metz,[17,18] for example, and so only a brief outline is given here. The method requires that the ob-

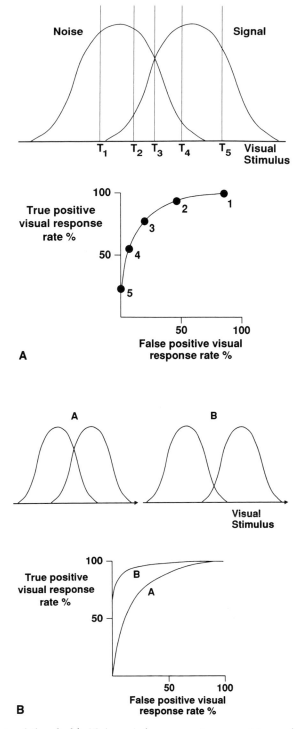

Fig. 1-5 (A) As the visual threshold, T, is varied, measured true-positive and false-positive response rates change, the threshold T_1 to T_5 producing points 1 to 5, respectively, on the ROC curve. **(B)** The ROC curve is generated by changes in the observer's decision criterion. Differences in effectiveness with which data are displayed, the separation between the signal and noise curves, are reflected by changes in the position of the corresponding ROC curve. Thus the technique permits one to distinguish between effects that are observer-dependent and those that are the result of better data presentation.

server should associate with his or her decision on whether an image is normal or abnormal a value indicating the degree of confidence in the response. Plotting the cumulative true- and false-positive response rates for each confidence category yields the ROC curve. What is being measured by the curve is the signal-to-noise ratio (SNR) for the particular task. The better the display, the higher the SNR associated with data displayed on it. Again, just how the SNR can be derived for a particular curve is beyond the discussion here, and the reader is referred to the literature.[17-19]

Also, the particular form of task has changed significantly. Although the type of task suitable for this analysis may vary widely, the basic paradigm is that it must involve the discrimination between two possible alternatives; the observer is only allowed to respond that the image belongs to either one class or the other (here referred to as noise or signal). This contrasts with the previous case, in which the signal intensity was systematically varied, with visual response being plotted as a function of signal intensity. Now the task may involve the use of normal and abnormal clinical images, a situation in which it is often impractical to measure signal intensity. All that is required is that the correct answer be known for each image used.

Ideal Observer

The imaging process can be regarded as having two stages, one involving detection and the other, data display.[20] Although the performance of a display requires a detailed understanding of human observers, the assessment of the quality of the acquired data can be performed in terms of the ideal observer.

The ideal observer is the Bayesian decision maker, which minimizes the cost or risk when determining a decision strategy for a given task. Given a suitable task, it is possible, subject to certain constraints, to calculate the SNR corresponding to the ideal

observer analyzing the acquired data. This value represents the best possible achievable SNR in any circumstances. Thus, we now can analyze imaging device performance in a fashion that is not dependent on the limitations of a human observer. Also we can investigate how well the performance of the human, using the displayed form of the data (i.e., the image), compares with the best achievable (i.e., the ideal observer analyzing the acquired data). A full description of the application of the ideal observer to a number of medical imaging modalities has been given by Wagner and Brown.[21]

However, this apparently perfect scenario has restrictions. The SNR for the ideal observer can, at present, be calculated only for a limited range of tasks; both the strategy and the form of the test images must be such that the number of possible alternatives is finite and well defined. Given known variability in the signal and background, a SNR can still be computed using a quasi-ideal rather than ideal-observer model.[22,23] However, although these limitations restrict the application of the approach to the more complex images and tasks representing clinical problems, the ideal-observer SNR can be calculated for the simple tasks often used to study device and display performance.

DISPLAY PERFORMANCE IN ULTRASOUND IMAGING

Relatively few attempts have been made to measure ultrasound image quality. The most comprehensive series of studies have been reported by Smith and Lopez and colleagues.[24-27] They made measurements of the threshold detectability of simulated lesions in speckle noise using the phantom shown in Figure 1-6A. The cones were made of different materials so that, when imaged, their contrast, C, differed. The conical shape meant that for any image plane, a set of circular lesions of varying contrast but constant diameter was displayed (Fig. 1-6B). By se-

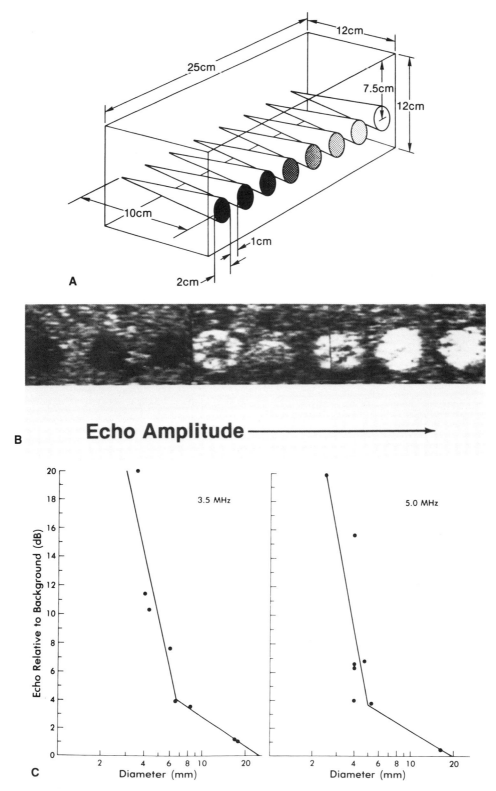

Fig. 1-6 (A) Phantom used to measure ultrasound image quality. **(B)** Example of image produced from this phantom. **(C)** Contrast-detail plot derived from observers viewing images of the phantom. (From Smith et al.,[24] with permission.)

lecting the image plane, the lesion diameter, d, could be altered.

The 50 percent true-positive visual response rate was chosen as defining the contrast needed for detection. The results were plotted as contrast-detail diagrams, similar to ones used for testing the performance of radiologic equipment,[28] a typical curve being shown in Figure 1-6C. This curve demonstrates that to detect objects comparable with the resolution of the system, high contrast is required, whereas for large lesions, contrast is strongly dependent on the lesion's size. The curve can be defined by the relationship Cd^n = constant, where $n = -2.3$ for small objects and $n = -0.33$ for large objects. Note that the small object relationship is similar to that found for other imaging modalities. A similarly shaped contrast-detail curve has been found using computer-simulated data.[29]

In their 1983 paper, Smith et al.[25] analyzed these results in terms of the performance of the ideal observer (i.e., the best possible performance achievable with the image data). For the purposes of the analysis, noise was treated as coherent speckle with a Rayleigh probability density function.[30] They demonstrated that for the small lesions, the performance of the real observer was less than that of the ideal, $Cd = \text{SNR}(S_{cx}S_{cz})^{1/2}$, S_{cx} and S_{cz} being the dimensions of the speckle correlation cell in the lateral and axial directions, respectively. The SNR being adopted by the human observers was found to have a value of 2.1 ± 0.6 and 1.99 ± 0.95 for the two scanners investigated. The relationship was similar to that for other noise-limited imaging modalities.

In a recent paper, Lopez et al.[27] looked at the errors inherent in the contrast-detail approach. In particular they were concerned that the SNR of the real observer was dependent on the decision threshold adopted by the observer. They found that the largest contribution to the error was due to the differences in the sensitivity attributed to the various observers. This, they suggested, might be due to the different degrees of experience acquired by the observers in carrying out the task. They concluded that "contrast-detail analysis may be impractical in a clinical environment, unless the observers are specifically and extensively trained in this task."

From the ideal-observer analysis, Smith et al.[25] concluded that there were at least four possible techniques for improving the detectability of low-contrast lesions (i.e., higher transducer frequencies, spatial compounding, broader bandwidth transducers, frequency compounding, and perhaps, image smoothing). The effect of image smoothing has been studied by Loupas et al.[31] They used a weighted median filter in which the weighting coefficient at point (i,j) in the 11×11 filter array was given by

$$w_{ij} = 99\frac{1 - 10s}{(\text{SNR})^2}$$

where s is the distance of point (i,j) from the center of the filter window and SNR is the ratio of the mean of all the terms in the window area to their standard deviation. This filter smooths without undue blurring of edges. The authors attempted no objective evaluation of the effect of filtering, simply commenting that on ultrasound abdominal images, the process "improves the detectability of subtle gray scale variations within the parenchyma, increases the visibility of small structures and seems to enhance the amount of information obtained from an image."

The effect of exposure level on image quality was studied by Harris et al.[32] Images of the liver and right kidney were made, as well as those of a phantom consisting of 0.3-mm nylon fibers and 0.75-cm-diameter anechoic "cysts" embedded in a mixture of gel and powdered graphite. The quality of the images was judged subjectively. They concluded that increasing the exposure level produced no obvious improvement in the diagnostic information. This, they conjectured, was because the SNR required to extract the relevant information was already so high that any reduction caused by lowering the exposure was not sufficient to prevent all the relevant information from being extracted from the image. However, they accepted that this might not be true in all cases; for example, the expected masking of the speckle pattern by electronic noise was observed in the phantom, and the depth at which it occurred was a function of exposure level.

Texture

Image texture measurements in ultrasound have received much attention. As they are considered separately in Chapter 5, they will not be discussed in detail here. However, work has been completed on comparing the performance of human observers with that of computers in classifying images according to texture. The human visual system is good at distinguishing changes in first-order statistics but, without at least detailed scrutiny, cannot perceive differences caused by third-order statistics. Second-order statistical differences fall into an intermediate category, with a range of tasks that the human performs with low efficiency. It is the second-order statistics (in the form of the noise power spectrum), however, that determine how readily lesions can be detected as well as play a part in tissue characterization.[33]

Garra et al.[34] compared a computer-based analysis of the texture of ultrasound liver images with the performance of human observers. Four tissue characterization parameters were considered: the frequency-dependent attenuation coefficient, the average distance between regularly positioned specular scatters, the ratio of specular to diffuse backscatter intensities, and a measure of the variability in the specular component normalized by the diffuse contribution. Both the performance of the computer analysis and that of the humans were measured using ROC curves. For patients with chronic hepatitis, the computer did significantly better than the humans, but for Gaucher's disease they performed equally well.

Coding of Intensity Information

The use of a gray scale to represent the intensity information in ultrasound images (Fig. 1-1) is widely adopted, although a few systems offer the option of false colors. There are two principal reasons why false-color intensity coding might be of value: to increase the effectiveness of the intensity scale by, for example, extending its dynamic range; and to distinguish between different types of information in the image.

One of the most widely used color scales is the "hot body," first proposed for coding ultrasound images.[35] In this the intensity scale varies from black through shades of red to white hot (Plate 1-2). Thus, as well as an increase in intensity being represented by a change in luminance or brightness, changes in color, or chromaticity, provide an extra dimension. Chan and Pizer[36] described a simple system for converting the video output from the scan converter circuit so that the image appears on a standard color television, coded as the hot-body spectrum.

In contrast to these scales, colors can be deliberately chosen to emphasize the difference between one intensity step and the next. In Plate 1-2, the colors have been selected to contrast with each other while still showing some natural progression from low-intensity blue to high-intensity red. Toma et al.[37] described a microcomputer-based system that produced high-resolution false-color ultrasound images in real-time.

The dynamic range of an intensity scale has

been measured by the number of perceptually different intensity levels in the scale. Using this measure, the contrasting color type of scale has been shown to have a greater dynamic range than the hot-body spectrum, with the gray scale having the smallest range.[38]

Apart from the potential for extending the dynamic range of the intensity scale, consideration must be given to ensuring that the chosen scale does not distort the intensity information, making it easier to perceive changes between display levels in one part of the scale than another. With this problem in mind, De Valk et al.[39] suggested a method for generating a color scale in which equal-sized steps up the scale produced equally well-perceived changes in chromaticity. One version of this scale is shown in Plate 1-2.

The gray scale also requires careful definition. Measurements of the density between the steps on a gray scale on commercial displays show that they can differ significantly. An approach to producing a perceptually linear scale has been described,[40] although it is not suggested that this might be the most effective way of assigning gray levels to image signal strength. There is also the question of how many gray levels are required to represent an image adequately. As so often with this sort of question, the answer depends on the type of image, in particular the amount of image noise and its spatial structure, and the task for which the image is to be used. Pizer and Chan[40] assessed the number of perceptible differences associated with intensity scales by measuring the minimum perceived brightness differences between the images of two noise-free rectangles. The results were 84 for a gray scale compared with 121 for a hot-body scale. However, this experiment did not involve any element of image structure in the task. Pratt[41] stated that 64 gray levels produce good quality images, whereas 32 give moderate quality. However, the introduction of noise reduces the number of gray levels judged to be necessary. Little

work has been performed with ultrasound images, but typically, displays use about 32 gray levels.

Sanders[42] studied the differences resulting from using either a white background display (positive image) or one with a black background (negative image). He concluded that when abnormalities are to be seen against an echogenic background (e.g., kidney and liver), they are best presented in the negative format, whereas structures with well-visualized boundaries (e.g., biliary tree and pancreas) appear clearer with a white background. Caution is required when interpreting these results, as image quality was assessed in a highly subjective fashion, using only a single observer. It was also necessary to increase the gain to obtain a "satisfactory" image when the positive display format was used. However, it does suggest that this is an aspect of display presentation that might benefit from further investigation.

Although color has advantages for intensity representation, it does have the drawback that it may introduce artificial contours into the image, particularly when adjacent color levels are perceptually distinct, and so distort spatial information. This is exacerbated if the chosen color sequence does not follow some "natural" order in which successive colors in the scale obviously represent an increase (or decrease) in intensity. In this case, there is a problem in identifying structure in an image, a lack of "associability."[43]

Crowe et al.,[44] using nuclear medicine images, showed that small changes in image intensity are best demonstrated with the contrasting color scale but also that this scale was the worst in a task involving spatial information. Scales such as that proposed by De Valk et al.[39] appeared to offer the best compromise.

The question of choice of intensity scale may appear somewhat academic when the operator has control over image intensity and contrast and the image data can be interrogated interactively. However, given the limited time available to the operator to make adjustments, an optimized intensity scale makes it more likely that all the available information is extracted from an image.

The second application of color to medical images is in its use for displaying additional information. The classic example of this is in Doppler (Plate 1-1), where flow information is shown in color superimposed on the standard B-mode image. The particular choice of colors depends on the information to be presented. When quantitative data are to be displayed, with color level being numerically related to some parameter, a contrasting scale offers the best solution. If the data are semiquantitative and the intention is to present an impression of the magnitudes of the parameter, the variation in hue is best. In Doppler, the choice of colors is a combination of the need to show both flow velocity and flow direction.

FUTURE DEVELOPMENTS

So far as the technical development of ultrasound display systems is concerned, the routine use of truly digital systems, with a full range of image processing facilities, would appear to be the next obvious stage of development. For reasons already given, this would be dependent on such systems being cheap and effectively acting in real-time.

Little work has been performed on the measurement of the effectiveness with which data are presented; this is a situation not limited to ultrasound imaging, although the way in which ultrasound images are interrogated leads to particular problems. The approach using signal detection theory appears to offer the greatest potential. It has two advantages: First, it allows the effectiveness with which data are displayed to be judged independently from observer behavior. Second, the quality

of the acquired data can, in certain circumstances, be measured without the need to perform lengthy perceptual experiments; the best possible achievable SNR can be computed, giving a gold standard for device performance assessment. It may be that in the future, assessment of the quality of ultrasound image data will be based on machine reading rather than involving the human observer.[24]

REFERENCES

1. Warwick R, Williams PL (eds): Gray's Anatomy. 35th Ed. Longman, Edinburgh, 1973
2. Stiles WH, Crawford BH: The luminous efficiency of rays entering the eye pupil at different points. Proc R Soc Lond [Biol] 112:428, 1933
3. Livingstone M, Hubel D: Segregation of form, color, movement, and depth: anatomy, physiology and perception. Science 240:740, 1988
4. Boynton RM: Human Color Vision. Holt, Rinehart & Winston, New York, 1979
5. Hering E: Outlines of a Theory of the Light Sense, 1877. Harvard University Press, Cambridge, 1964
6. de Valois RL, de Valois KK: Neural coding of color. p. 117. In Carterette EC, Friedmann NP (eds): Handbook of Perception. Academic Press, New York, 1975
7. Land EH: The retinex theory of color vision. Sci Am 237:108, 1977
8. Dainty JC, Shaw R: Image Science. Academic Press, London, 1974
9. Campbell FW, Kulikowski JJ, Levinson J: The effect of orientation on the visual resolution of gratings. J Physiol (Lond) 187:427, 1966
10. Campbell FW, Maffei L: Contrast and spatial frequency. Sci Am 231:106, 1974
11. Campbell FG, Green DG: Optical and retinal factors affecting visual resolution. J Physiol (Lond) 181:576, 1956
12. Cornsweet TN: Visual Perception. Academic Press, New York, 1970
13. Pitt WR, Sharp PF, Chesser RB, Dendy PP: Radionuclide image minification can compensate for coarse digitization. J Nucl Med 24:1046, 1983

14. Kelly DH: Visual responses to time dependent stimuli. I. Amplitude sensitivity measurements. J Opt Soc Am 51:422, 1961

15. Murch GM: Visual and Auditory Perception. Bobbs-Merrill, New York, 1973

16. Tanner WP, Swets JA: A decision-making theory of visual detection. Psychol Rev 61: 401, 1954

17. Metz CE: ROC methodology in radiologic imaging. Invest Radiol 21:720, 1986

18. Metz CE: Some practical issues of experimental design and data analysis in radiological ROC studies. Invest Radiol 24:234, 1989

19. Green DM, Swets JA: Signal Detection Theory and Psychophysics. Wiley, New York, 1964

20. Wagner RF, Brown DG, Pastel MS: The application of information theory to the assessment of computed tomography. Med Phys 6: 83, 1979

21. Wagner RF, Brown DG: Unified SNR analysis of medical imaging systems. Phys Med Biol 30:489, 1985

22. Fiete RD, Barrett HH, Smith WE, Myers KJ: Hotelling trace criterion and its correlation with human-observer performance. J Opt Soc Am [A]4:945, 1987

23. Myers KJ, Wagner RF: Detection of estimation: human vs ideal performance as a function of information. SPIE Med Imaging II 914:291, 1988

24. Smith SW, Lopez H: A contrast-detail analysis of diagnostic ultrasound imaging. Med Phys 9:4, 1982

25. Smith SW, Wagner RF, Sandrick JM, Lopez H: Low contrast detectability and contrast/detail analysis in medical ultrasound. IEEE Trans Sonics Ultrason 30:164, 1983

26. Smith SW, Lopez H, Bodine WJ: Frequency independent ultrasound contrast-detail analysis. Ultrasound Med Biol 11:467, 1985

27. Lopez H, Loew MH, Butler PF et al: A clinical evaluation of contrast-detail analysis for ultrasound images. Med Phys 17:48, 1990

28. Cohen G: Contrast-detail-dose analysis of six different computed tomographic scanners. J Comp Assist Tomog 3:197, 1979

29. Lowe H, Bamber JC, Webb S, Cook-Martin G: Perceptual studies of contrast, texture and detail in ultrasound B-scans. SPIE Med Imaging II 914:40, 1988

30. Wagner RF, Smith SW, Sandrik JM, Lopez H: Statistics of speckle in ultrasound B-scans. IEEE Trans Sonics Ultrason 30:156, 1983

31. Loupas T, McDicken WN, Allan PL: Noise reduction in ultrasonic images by digital filtering. Br J Radiol 60:389, 1987

32. Harris GR, Stewart HF, Leo FP, Sanders RC: Relationship between image quality and ultrasound exposure level in diagnostic US devices. Radiology 173:313, 1989

33. Wagner RF, Insana MF, Brown DG: Progress in signal and texture discrimination in medical imaging. SPIE Applications Opt Instrumentation Med XII 535:57, 1985

34. Garra BS, Insana MF, Shawker TH et al: Quantitative ultrasonic detection and classification of diffuse liver disease. Comparison with human observer performance. Invest Radiol 24:196, 1989

35. Milan J, Taylor KJW: The application of the temperature scale to ultrasound imaging. J Clin Ultrasound 3:171, 1975

36. Chan FH, Pizer SM: An ultrasonogram display system using a natural color scale. J Clin Ultrasound 4:335, 1976

37. Toma SK, Seeds JW, Cefalo RC: High-resolution computerized color transformation of real-time gray scale ultrasound images. J Clin Ultrasound 17:353, 1989

38. Pizer SM, Zimmerman JB, Johnston RE: Concepts of the display of medical images. IEEE Trans Nucl Sci 29:1322, 1982

39. De Valk JPJ, Epping WJM, Heringa A: Colour representation of biomedical data. Med Biol Eng Comput 23:343, 1985

40. Pizer SM, Chan FH: Evaluation of the number of discernible levels produced by a display. p. 561. In Di Paola R, Khan E (eds): Information Processing in Medical Imaging. INSERM, Paris, 1980

41. Pratt WK: Digital Image Processing. Wiley, New York, 1978

42. Sanders RC: Comparison between black and white backgrounds for ultrasonic images. J Clin Ultrasound 8:413, 1980

43. Cormack J, Hutton B: Minimisation of data transfer losses in the display of digitised scintigraphic images. Phys Med Biol 25:271, 1980

44. Crowe EJ, Sharp PF, Undrill PE, Ross PGB: Effectiveness of colour in displaying radionuclide images. Med Biol Eng Comput 26: 57, 1988

2

Probes as Used in Cardiology With Emphasis on Transesophageal and Intravascular Applications

Nicolaas Bom
Pieter D. Brommersma
Charles T. Lancée

Many cardiovascular ultrasound transducers are being used over a wide frequency range in cardiology (Fig. 2-1). The transthoracic diagnostic applications are in the frequency range below 5 MHz, whereas transesophageal and epicardial applications use frequencies in the range of 3 to 12 MHz. The intracardiac catheter tip system operates at intermediate frequencies of about 12 MHz and is a low-frequency large-size version of the 20- to 30-MHz high-frequency catheter tip intravascular devices.[1]

It is well known that the beam directivity depends on the wavelength and the active acoustic surface of the probe. For the non-invasive applications, the probe size must be, and can be, larger compared with the applications at the high-frequency range. However, the attenuation of ultrasound in tissue increases with increased frequency. Thus, the maximum scan depth depends on the frequency. With increasing frequency, both lateral and axial resolutions improve. In practice, it is apparent that a compromise be-

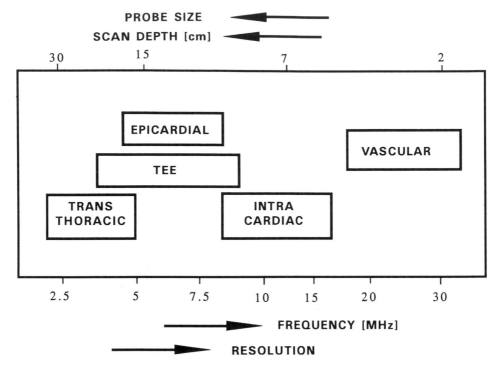

Fig. 2-1 Frequency range for probes as used in cardiac and vascular imaging. TEE, transesophageal echocardiography. (From Bom and Roelandt,[1] with permission.)

tween the limitation in scan depth and the desired resolution must be obtained. With this in mind, we can see that the indicated application areas and the corresponding required scan depth in Figure 2-1 show a logical distribution over the frequency range.

In the early days of real-time cardiac imaging, the linear array[1a] approach was used. This principle can be described as the rapid sequential use of adjacent subgroups of elements from a long strip of small individual elements. This method resulted in a rectangular image format, but because of the large footprint of the transducer, the method showed limited applicability for transthoracic imaging of the heart, where point entry between the ribs appeared to be required. Therefore, in cardiology, several different sector scanners became the method of choice.

In sector scanners, beam steering can be per-

formed in two ways. The transducer or a mirror can be mechanically rotated or pivoted. In the phased array principle as first described by Somer,[2] acoustic energy from a small linear array is used by activating all the single elements with different delay lines to create an acoustic beam under a given angle. This method can be quickly repeated to cover a complete sectorial cross section through the tissue. For most applications in transthoracic, transesophageal, and epicardial use in cardiology today, the phased array sector scan principle is used. It combines the possibilities for a small footprint with the electronic flexibility to use different focusing points in transmission and dynamic focusing in reception, thereby improving the resolution. However, dynamic focusing can only take place in the image plane, the lateral direction. Transverse focusing is achieved with an acoustic (fixed) lens. A disadvantage of the phased array is the decrease in sensitivity when steering angles become larger: this is due to the projected aperture of the active acoustic area. This disadvantage is not present in mechanical sector scanners, where, in addition, with today's annular array technology, focusing in both the transverse and the lateral direction is available. However, phased arrays have no mechanical motion and therefore are more reliable in practical use. Phased arrays are also compact in size and for this reason are the method of choice for applications where size becomes a limiting factor, such as in the transesophageal approach.

EARLY INTRALUMINAL IMAGING

Already very early in the history of diagnostic ultrasound, echo information was used to form a cross-sectional image (Fig. 2-2). For this purpose, the acoustic beam had to be scanned through the cross-sectional plane. To obtain a realistic display, the acoustic beam direction and beam deflection on the display had to be synchronized. Mechani-

cally rotated transducers were used such as the one described by Wild and Reid[3] in 1955 for rectal tumor localization.

Omoto[4] described an intravenous catheter approach in 1962 with guide wire tip to study cardiac structures, and Ebina et al.[5] described a miniature concave transducer for rotation inside a rubber cuff in the esophagus in 1964. Wells[6] described an intravenous device with flexible shaft and rotating mirror in 1965 for cross-sectional imaging of veins. Eggleton et al.[7] approximated a cardiac cross section by rotating a four-element catheter. Results of his system depended on a stable state of the heart because they accumulated data over many beats for reconstruction of a cross-section in a selected steady state. In 1971, Bom et al.[8] reported a two-dimensional real-time phased array ultrasound imaging catheter, which comprised a 32-element circular array with an outer diameter of 3.2 mm mounted at the tip of a 9-French catheter (Fig. 2-3). The final design was chosen to operate at a frequency of 5.6 MHz with a narrow main beam. With this catheter, real-time intraluminal images such as left ventricular cross

Wild	1955	echo-endoscope	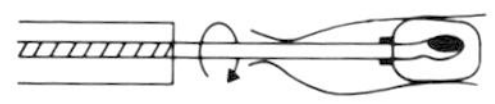	rectal tumour location
Omoto	1962	rotating probe C-scan	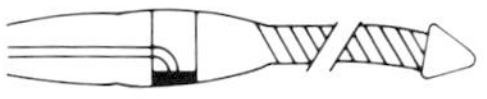	intracardiac tomography
Ebina	1964	transesophageal P.P.I. scanning	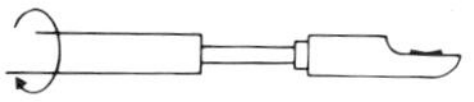	heart and vessels
Wells	1965	rotating mirror	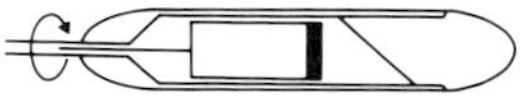	intravenous
Eggleton	1969	4-elements e.c.g. triggered	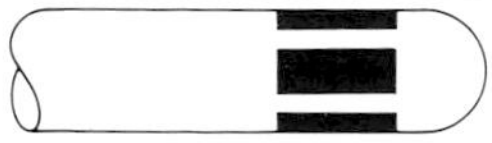	heart
Bom	1971	32-elements cylindrical phased array	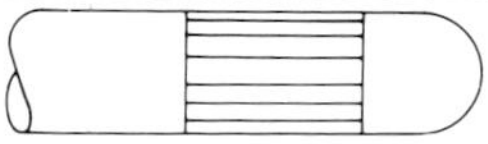	intracardiac tomography

Fig. 2-2 Chronologic order of examples of intraluminal imaging systems as described by several authors.

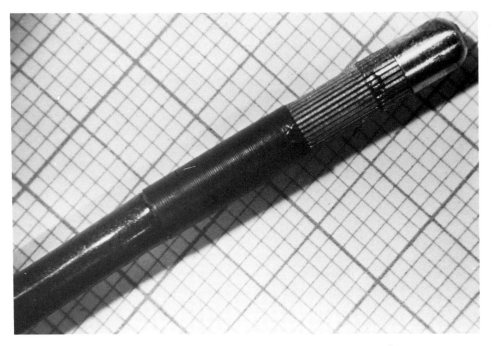

Fig. 2-3 Phased array 32-element catheter as described by Bom et al.[8] in early 1970s.

sections were recorded in the early 1970s. The rationale for these intraluminal approaches was to bring the probe close to, if not into, the organ to be studied.

A two-dimensional imaging system to study the heart from nearby through the esophagus was described by Hisanaga et al. in 1977.[9] The scanning device consisted of a rotating single element in a liquid-filled balloon mounted at the tip of a gastroscope. In 1980 DiMagno et al.[10] described a high-frequency linear array for small parts scanning. The electronic phased array esophageal transducer was described by Souquet et al.[11] in 1982 and operated at a frequency of 2.25 MHz. From this moment on, phased array scanning through the esophagus rapidly evolved. In our institute, a first design with a 24-element 3.1-MHz array was described by Lancée et al,[12] also in 1982. Improvements in microminiature cutting and bonding technology resulted in a series of transducers with progressively better image quality. A 52-ele-

ment 4.7-MHz array with a pitch of 210 μm was introduced and reported by de Jong et al.[13] The final design was a 64-element 5.6-MHz array with a pitch of only 160 μm. It was reported by de Jong et al. in 1985.[14]

WHY TRANSESOPHAGEAL ECHOCARDIOGRAPHY?

Transthoracic *precordial* echocardiography is a unique method for noninvasive study of cardiac morphology and function. The two-dimensional technique is ideally suited to visualize cardiac geometry, whereas accurate measurement of, for example, left ventricular wall thickness is best obtained from M-mode recordings guided by two-dimensional cross-sectional echo. With the introduction of pulsed, continuous-wave, and color Doppler, study of the velocity of the blood flow also became possible. The advantage of two-dimensional precordial echography is that the transducer can be in different positions on the chest wall, using several acoustic windows. This results in a large number of spatial orientations for interrogating planes of diagnostic crosssections. In daily practice, precordial cardiac ultrasound equipment has become the workhorse of the cardiologist.

The rationale for *transesophageal* echocardiography (TEE) is that this technique overcomes many of the disadvantages experienced with the precordial approach. Because the esophagus lies next to the heart without interfering structures in between, little signal attenuation occurs. This allows the use of higher-frequency transducers. Thus, high resolution and detailed images can be achieved. Structures in the far-field of a precordial transducer are anatomically close to the transesophageal transducer. Other limitations of precordial echocardiography such

as the presence of bone and lung tissue can be avoided.

EXAMPLE OF AN ADULT TEE PROBE

As already described, the phased array technology seems optimal for application to TEE probes in the frequency range of the instruments of today. The active probe surface is usually a rectangular-shaped piezoelectric slab, which is cut into small individual elements. For steering of the acoustic beam, all these elements are used in concert with different delays. Therefore the elements are individually connected by a multiwire cable through the gastroscope pipe to the echo machine. The size of the wires has decreased greatly in the past 10 years, which offered the possibility to miniaturize the probes. Di-

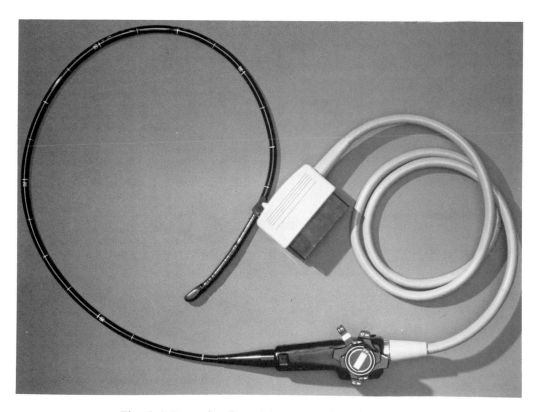

Fig. 2-4 Example of an adult transesophageal transducer.

mensional parameters of an example such as the 64-element 5.6–MHz TEE probe are as follows. The gastroscope pipe diameter is 10 mm; the aperture of the array is 9×10 mm^2; the total tip width/height is 14/10 mm. This example of a transesophageal phased array transducer is shown in Figure 2-4.

The tip can be angulated in two perpendicular planes by two pairs of Bowden cables connected to knobs at the proximal end of the TEE probe. It must be considered at this point that observations can be made only in a scan plane perpendicular to the length axis of the gastroscopic pipe because of orientation of the elements in the phased array.

PEDIATRIC AND BIPLANE TEE PROBES

Although children normally are scanned from the chest with sufficient image quality, there are circumstances when TEE would be preferable, especially after surgical procedures in which the chest had been opened. The previously described transesophageal probe is made for use in adults, and it is too large to be applied in small children. Therefore a smaller version was developed. The size reduction was obtained by reduction of the number of elements to 48. The total array width became 8 mm, which allows a tip width of 10 mm. The multiwire electric cable could be reduced accordingly. Further reduction of the shaft diameter was obtained by use of only one pair of Bowden cables, which reduced the tip manipulation to up–down motion. This resulted in a shaft diameter of 7 mm. As stated before, with a fixed phased array construction at the tip of the gastroscope pipe, only a "fixed" diagnostic plane can be selected. This is a limitation.

An important expansion of the cross section's selectability is made with a TEE probe that has two arrays in its tip, one for the "standard" transverse images and one to make longitudinal cross sections. It is possible to switch between the two arrays when the probe is inserted in the patient. Because the arrays are placed next to each other, there may be a contact problem after switching; the probe must then be repositioned.

For two arrays, the cable diameter will increase. Luckily this development fell together with further miniaturization of the wires, so that today the 18-wire cable needed for a 2×64-elements biplane probe has almost the same outer diameter as the old 64-wire cable!

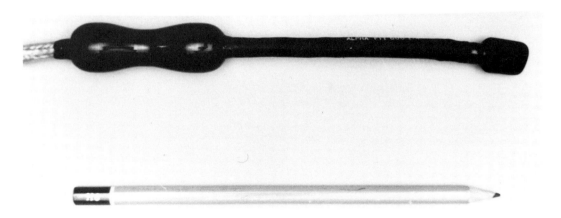

Fig. 2-5 Surgical hand-held probe based on TEE technology.

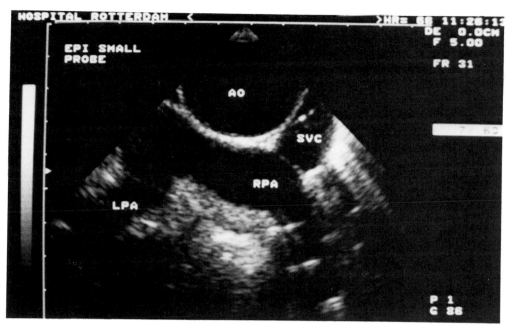

Fig. 2-6 Cross section recorded from ascending aorta. This view demonstrates bifurcation of pulmonary trunk and includes superior vena cava. LPA, left pulmonary artery; RPA, right pulmonary artery; SVC, superior vena cava.

SURGICAL PROBES

High-quality ultrasound images can be obtained during cardiac surgery by placing a transducer directly on the heart. These images can be used to validate the indications before the operation and used afterward to check the results of the surgical procedure. Sector scanners are the most effective for scanning the beating heart because of their small contact area. A small probe consisting of just an array on a cable was built under the name *fingertip probe*. The surgeon was supposed to hold the array in his or her fingers or fasten it to his or her finger with tape. This approach turned out to be unsuccessful. Subsequently a new "fingertip probe plus handle" was developed. This version incorporated a stiff, yet bendable shaft between the array and a handle. This allows the surgeon to set the shaft as he or she requires and

to place it anywhere next to and on the heart. This probe is illustrated in Figure 2-5. An example of a cardiac cross section as obtained with this surgical probe is shown in Figure 2-6.

VARIOPLANE TEE

Biplane scanning already improved the imaging possibilities of TEE. However, a further expansion of the possibly available cross sections can be achieved if the array is rotatable in the tip. This allows an optimal search for the diagnostic views. The idea was described by Schlüter et al. in 1982,[15] but technical problems delayed the appearance of a device for almost 10 years. These problems included the connections for the array; the mechanism to rotate the array; and how to avoid moving parts at the surface, or when

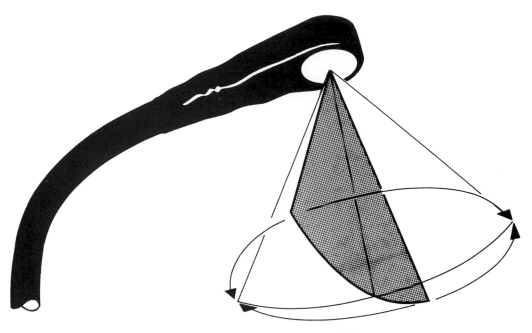

Fig. 2-7 Varioplane TEE principle.

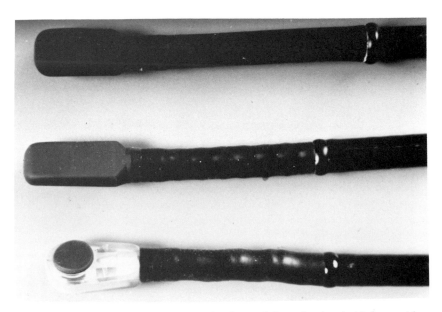

Fig. 2-8 Three generations of TEE probes: single-plane adult probe **(top)**; biplane with a transverse and a longitudinal array in its tip **(middle)**; varioplane probe **(bottom)**.

a construction with moving parts at the surface is chosen, the sealing.

The endoscope steering house has two knobs, normally used to move the tip in the up–down and left–right directions. In the varioplane device, the tip motion is limited to the up–down movement. The left–right flexibility is frozen and the second knob is used to rotate the array. The scan head of the varioplane transducer consists of a 5-MHz phased array. This offers the possibility to view the (standard) transverse cross section, the (biplane) longitudinal cross-section, and all the planes in between. A schematic drawing of its possibilities is shown in Figure 2-7.

The design was judged on two major parameters: tip size and image quality. These should be close to those of the gold standard, the single-plane adult probe. To achieve the same image quality, 64 elements are required. However, the usual array configuration is rectangular. For a 64-element array with a center frequency of 5 MHz, this results in a 9 × 10-mm rectangle. If this array is used for a varioplane construction, this would lead to a total tip width of about 17 mm, which was believed to be unacceptable. To achieve an acceptable tip size, the rectangular shape is changed into an octagon. Measurements on the acoustic beam profile of the octagonal shape show little change of the main lobe. The transverse side-lobe level decreased, which improved the image quality. The total width of the tip with the octagon array can be kept at 15 mm. Transverse focusing is achieved with an acoustic lens that covers the array. The varioplane prototype is illustrated in Figure 2-8; the beam pattern is shown in Figure 2-9.

HIGHER FREQUENCY

As pointed out before, resolution and depth of field are closely related to frequency. An improvement in resolution by increase in frequency always decreases the scan depth. However, for pediatric echocardiography and especially TEE, a very short range is needed. Frequencies up to 7.5 MHz should be able to view the total heart of a newborn. This higher frequency also allows the construction of a very small probe. The element width for a 7.5-MHz phased array is only 100 μm (one-half wavelength in water). A group of 10 elements has a total width of 1 mm! Arrays of these dimensions require careful treatment and are difficult to connect. Prototypes are being made and show detailed structures of the heart but over a limited depth.

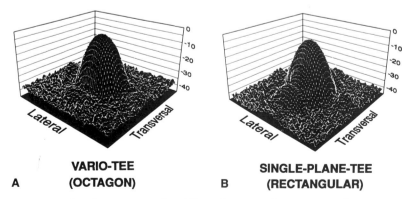

| A | VARIO-TEE (OCTAGON) | B | SINGLE-PLANE-TEE (RECTANGULAR) |

Fig. 2-9 Beam pattern plot for octagon plot (**A**) and rectangular active surface (**B**) as used in the TEE varioplane.

With the increased use of interventional techniques in vascular therapy, it became clear that more information on the vascular wall and its pathology is needed. Intravascular imaging techniques that operate in the 20- to 40-MHz range provide information on the arterial wall. This information becomes mandatory in the application of the newer generation of interventional devices, both in cardiology and in radiology. In intravascular ultrasound imaging, minute transducers are mounted at the tip of a catheter.

For intravascular ultrasound imaging systems, piezoelectric elements with an active acoustic surface in the order of 1 mm^2 are used. Only in combination with frequencies such as 30 MHz can a sufficiently narrow acoustic beam profile be obtained. For intravascular imaging, the axial resolution is in the order of 0.1 mm, and in the lateral direction, it is in the order of 0.3 to 0.5 mm.[1] In Figure 2-10, the penetration depth in blood, defined as the −20-dB level measured in reflection as function of frequency, is illustrated. For frequencies used in intravascular imaging, the penetration depth is rather small. For intracardiac catheters, a low-frequency version (about 12 MHz) of the intravascular technology is adopted, as was indicated previously. In this frequency range, TEE starts to divert into technologies used for vascular imaging.

PRINCIPLES OF INTRAVASCULAR IMAGING SYSTEMS

Recent intravascular ultrasound echo systems are based either on a mechanically rotated acoustic element or on electronically switched elements.[17] These systems provide a real-time cross-sectional image of the artery.

Rotating Element

In Figure 2-11A, the rotating tip system is illustrated schematically. The shaft (1) must be very flexible. It contains the electric wires for the transducer. The element (3) is positioned in such a way that no transmission pulse effect appears on the display because the echo travel time to the dome (2) is of sufficient duration. It allows imaging very close to the catheter outer wall because no "dead zone" or transient effect is present. The dome must be acoustically transparent.

Rotating Mirror

The rotating mirror technique is similar to the previously described method. Schematically, this method is shown in Figure 2-11B. The flexible shaft (1), the transparent dome (2), and the echo transducer (3) are assembled with a mirror (4). Because of the nonmoving transducer, rotating electric wires are avoided. Acoustic lenses and focusing shapes of the mirror have been described elsewhere.[17]

Electronically Switched Phased Array

The catheter shown in Figure 2-11C contains many small acoustic elements (2), which are positioned cylindrically around the catheter

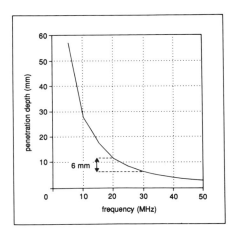

Fig. 2-10 Penetration depth as function of frequency. (From Bom et al.,[16] with permission.)

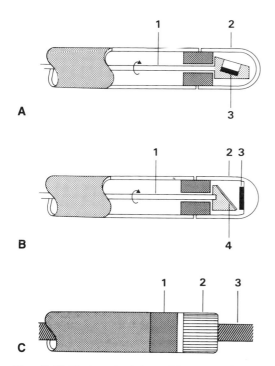

Fig. 2-11 Basic principles of intravascular imaging methods. (From Bom et al.,[18] with permission.)

tip. The number of elements may be any practical number, such as 32 or 64. The tip may contain an electronic component (1) to reduce the number of electrically conductive wires. The construction allows a central guide wire for easy insertion of the catheter (3). The electronically switched phased array catheter system has been referred to earlier.[8] By introduction of time delays, subgroups of elements together may form a "single larger echo transducer." This process can be repeated sequentially with adjacent subgroups by electronic switching and yields real-time imaging.

The same type of transducer can be used with a different kind of image processing. In this arrangement, each individual small element is used as a transmitter. The reflected signals

are received by all elements. This information is stored; then, information from all single elements is used together for real-time image reconstruction.

SOME LIMITATIONS

With mechanically rotated systems, the drive shaft must be very flexible, whereas the torsional rigidity must be large. Angle variations between both ends create artifacts in the image. With the phased array systems, either the multiple wires cause a problem or an electronic switching circuit has to be built in the catheter tip. In all events, the positioning of the active acoustic surface at the outer boundary creates an acoustic dead zone. This and possible artifacts caused by the rotational drive shaft in mechanically rotated systems are current limitations.

SOME EXAMPLES AND FUTURE DIRECTIONS

Intravascular studies have shown that from the echo appearance, artery morphology can be distinguished.[19] Muscular arteries have a hypoechoic smooth muscle component in the media, which results in a three-layered appearance. The bright inner layer represents the intima and the internal elastic lamina, the echo-poor intermediate layer represents the media, and the bright external layer represents the adventitia. The walls of elastic arteries and veins have a more homogeneous appearance.

In Figure 2-12, two intravascular cross sections are shown before balloon dilatation in the femoral artery. At position A, where the hypoechoic media is clearly visible in an area with still a large open lumen, a circumferential deposit is also visible, together with the echo catheter. Cross section B shows the center of the narrowing indicated in the left panel of the figure, where almost no open lumen

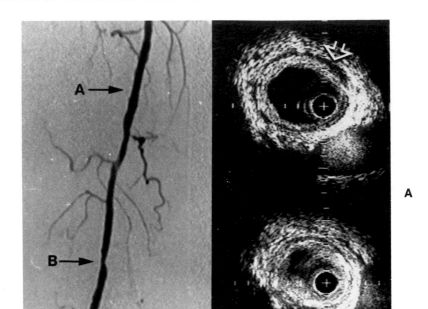

Fig. 2-12 Angiogram **(left panel)** reveals a 50 percent stenosis of right superficial femoral artery. Intravascular ultrasound images **(A, B)** are from positions indicated in angiogram. Proximally a large lumen is imaged with diffuse intimal thickening (1 mm). The dark layer corresponds with the media (open arrow). The femoral vein is noted at the 5-o'clock position. At the level of stenosis **(B)**, the medial layer is visible between the 11- and 6-o'clock positions. Evidence of calcium deposition causing shadowing is seen at the 7-o'clock position (solid arrow). Calibration markers are 1 mm. (Courtesy of W. J. Gussenhoven.)

is present, and because of ingrowth, also anechoic media disappearance from the image. The solid arrow indicates a small calcified area identified by high echo density and the shadow zone behind it at greater depth. Note that in frame A, the cross section from an adjacent vein is visible with the blood as an apparent spontaneous echo contrast in the center.[20]

As already indicated, it is possible to explore the heart with lower frequency and thus deeper penetrating ultrasound. Pandian et al.[21] described a mechanically rotating 12.5-MHz ultrasound catheter, the results of which are illustrated in Figure 2-13. The intracardiac echo images show short axis views of the left ventricle obtained during diastole

(left) and systole (right). Pandian et al. reported that in experimental studies it was found that such low-frequency catheters could demonstrate abnormalities such as tears or avulsion of the aortic valve cusps, pericardial effusion, and ventricular dysfunction.

When considering future directions, a number of catheters that combine intraluminal ultrasound and various forms of balloon angioplasty must be mentioned. A survey of many of these ideas has been made by Crowley et al.[22] An example is indicated in Figure 2-14, illustrating a combination device as used for animal studies and early human clinical trials. Whereas the higher frequencies used in the transesophageal approach allow

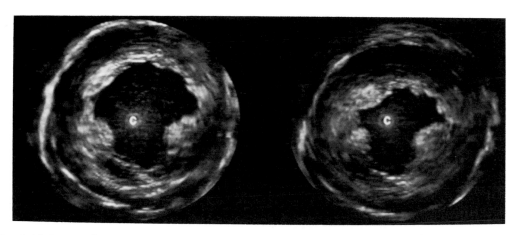

Fig. 2-13 Intracardiac echo images of the left ventricle in its short axis obtained with a 12.5-MHz ultrasound catheter positioned at the center of the ventricle clearly delineate the left ventricular cavity during diastole **(left)** and systole **(right)**. (From Pandian et al.,[21] with permission. Courtesy of N. Pandian.)

better resolution and more specific diagnostic information to be obtained, this tendency is even more apparent in the high-frequency intravascular area. Not only does the combination with interventional therapeutic devices become possible, but also tissue identification may become practical in this frequency area. As an example of the latter possibility, de Kroon et al.[23] described the angle dependence of backscatter power at 27 MHz from the arterial vessel wall. Because of variations in the angle of incidence, significant variations in the backscatter were found in the intima, the muscular and the

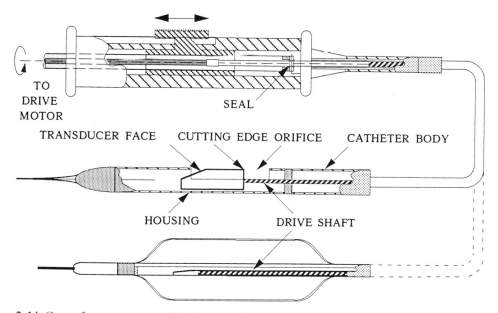

Fig. 2-14 One of many proposed devices combining ultrasound and interventional therapy. This instrument has an atherectomy device or, alternatively, a balloon. (From Crowley et al.,[22] with permission. Courtesy of B. Crowley.)

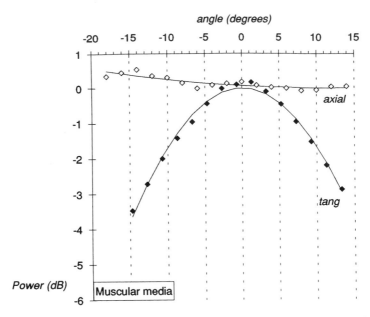

Fig. 2-15 Normalized power versus angle curve of muscular media of one specimen from a tangential and an axial scan. (From de Kroon et al.,[23] with permission. Courtesy of M. de Kroon.)

elastic media, the adventitia, and the external elastic lamina. For instance, the muscular media showed anisotropic behavior in angle dependence. This anisotropic behavior probably is caused by the dominant orientation of the elastin fibers in these tissues. Figure 2-15 illustrates the variation in backscattered power versus angle of incidence in the axial and tangential planes. This is just one example of new research areas that are being opened with the introduction of new high-frequency probes.

CONCLUSIONS

The past decade has shown a worldwide effort to improve the clinical value of cardiac ultrasound equipment. High frequency yields better resolution; however, the scan depth decreases proportionally. As a result, there is a tendency to combine the high-frequency approach with a more invasive technique to bring the transducer close to the structure to be studied. New miniaturization

technologies further allow echographic observation, even from inside small arteries. With these approaches, new diagnostic methods will appear, including new directions in tissue identification.

REFERENCES

1. Bom N, Roelandt JRTC: Intravascular ultrasound: newest branch on the echo-tree. Cardiovasc Imag 4:55, 1992
1a. Bom N: New Concepts in Echocardiography. Stenfert Kroese, Leyden, 1972
2. Somer JC: Electronic sector scanning for ultrasonic diagnosis. p. 37. Progress Report. Medisch Physisch Instituut, Utrecht, 1968
3. Wild JJ, Reid JM: Ultrasonic rectal endoscope for tumor location. Am Inst Ultrason Med 4: 59, 1955
4. Omoto R: Intracardiac scanning of the heart with the aid of ultrasonic intravenous probe. Jpn Heart J 8:569, 1967
5. Ebina T, Oka S, Tanaka M et al: The diagnostic application of ultrasound to the disease

in mediastinal organs. Ultrasono-tomography for the heart and great vessels. Sci Rep Res Inst Tohoku Univ 12:199, 1965

6. Wells PNT: Developments in medical ultrasonics. World Med Electron 4:272, 1966

7. Eggleton RC, Townsend C, Kossoff G et al: Computerised ultrasonic visualization of dynamic ventricular configurations. 8th ICMBE, Chicago, Session 10-3, 1969

8. Bom N, Lancée CT, van Egmond FC: An ultrasonic intracardiac scanner. Ultrasonics 10:72, 1972

9. Hisanaga K, Hisanaga A, Nagata K, Yoshida S: A new transesophageal real-time two-dimensional echocardiographic system using a flexible tube and its clinical application. Proc Jpn Soc Ultrason Med 32:43, 1977

10. DiMagno EP, Regan PT, Wilson DA et al: Ultrasonic endoscope. Lancet i:629, 1980

11. Souquet J, Hanrath P, Zitelli L et al: Transesophageal phased array for imaging the heart. IEEE Trans Biomed Eng 29:707, 1982

12. Lancée CT, Ligtvoet CM, de Jong N: On the design and construction of a transesophageal scanner. p. 260. In Hanrath P, Bleifeld W, Souquet J (eds): Cardiovascular Diagnosis by Ultrasound. Martinus Nijhoff, The Hague, 1982

13. de Jong N, Lancée CT, Gussenhoven WJ et al: Transesophageal echocardiography. Med Biol Eng Comput 23; Suppl 1; Proc XIV Int Conf Med Biol Eng & VII Int Conf Med Phys, Espoo: 204, 1985

14. de Jong N, Lancée CT, Gussenhoven WJ et al: Transesofagale echocardiografie. Ultrasonoor Bull 2:28, 1985

15. Schlüter M, Langenstein BA, Polster J et al: Transesophageal cross-sectional echocardiography with a phased array transducer system. Technique and initial clinical results. Br Heart J 48:67, 1982

16. Bom N, Lancée CT, Gussenhoven EJ et al: Basic principles of intravascular ultrasound imaging. p. 7. In Tobis JM, Yock PG (eds): Intravascular Ultrasound Imaging. Churchill Livingstone, New York, 1992

17. Hartley CJ, Sartori MP, Henry PD: Intravascular imaging with ultrasound. In: Microsensors and Catheter-Based Imaging Technology. SPIE 904:103, 1988

18. Bom N, ten Hoff H, Lancée CT et al: Early and recent intraluminal ultrasound devices. Int J Card Imaging 4:79, 1989

19. Gussenhoven WJ, Essed CE, Frietman P et al: Intravascular echographic assessment of vessel wall characteristics; a correlation with histology. Int J Card Imaging 4:105, 1989

20. Gussenhoven WJ, The SHK, Gerritsen P et al: Real-time intravascular ultrasonic imaging before and after balloon angioplasty. J Clin Ultrasound 19:294, 1991

21. Pandian NG, Schwartz SL, Weintraub AR et al: Intracardiac echography: current developments. Int J Card Imaging 6:207, 1991

22. Crowley RJ, Hamm MA, Joshi SH et al: Ultrasound guided therapeutic catheters: recent developments and clinical results. Int J Card Imaging 6:145, 1991

23. De Kroon MGM, Van der Wal LF, Gussenhoven WJ et al: Backscatter directivity and integrated backscatter power of arterial tissue. Int J Card Imaging 6:265, 1991

3

Ultrasound Contrast Agents

Barry B. Goldberg

Gramiak and Shah[1] in 1968 were the first to report on the introduction of a substance that increased the reflectivity of the blood. In patients with normal aortic valves who were undergoing ascending aortography, saline was injected through a catheter into the supravalvular region during continuous M-mode echocardiographic recording. The injected saline was detected as a cloud of echoes contained within the lumen of the aortic root. At the time, Gramiak and Shah speculated that the saline-produced echoes were arising from microbubbles of gas. Other investigators then used such solutions as indocyanine green to confirm the presence of such cardiac abnormalities as shunts and valvular insufficiency.[2,3] In 1971, using a suprasternal placement of an ultrasound transducer, I was able to confirm the vascular structures being imaged. By injection of a solution of indocyanine green through a catheter placed in these vessels, echoes were produced (Fig. 3-1).[4] This approach was also used to confirm that ultrasound could visualize the common bile duct.[5] The reflectivity of the injected solutions was caused by the presence of microbubbles of gas, which went back into solution over time.[6,7]

Since then, various other solutions have proved to be useful as ultrasound contrast agents by virtue of their ability to trap microbubbles. In fact, almost any solution that is agitated and then injected into a vein or artery produces echoes. The intensity of the echoes varies with the type of solution used, with the most viscous solutions containing the most gas bubbles.

EARLY WORK

Over the years, sonification of solutions, including dextrose, sorbitol, and renographin, has become the most common approach for the generation of ultrasound contrast material.[8] Most of the early work was performed to evaluate different cardiographic abnormalities. Gramiak and Shah used a contrast agent as an aid in identifying the aortic valve. Others used it to evaluate valvular regurgitation and to confirm the presence, as well as the size, of shunts at atrial and ventricular levels.[9,10] This initial research recorded the actual increase in echogenicity within the cavities. Recently, the same concept has been used with Doppler to

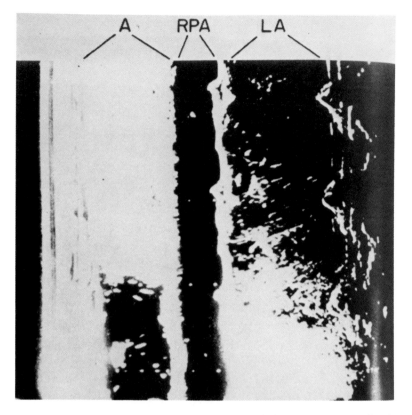

Fig. 3-1 Suprasternal M-mode ultrasound imaging obtained during injection of indocyanine green into left atrium. Typical snowlike echo pattern is first seen in left atrium (LA) followed by its appearance in the aorta (A). RPA, right pulmonary artery. (From Goldberg,[4] with permission.)

increase its signal strength.[11] This approach has helped to demonstrate more clearly cardiac shunts as well as flow reversals and to increase the ability to detect coronary artery blood flow.[12,13]

TYPES OF CONTRAST AGENTS

One of the problems with the solutions that use gas bubbles formed principally by means of agitation was that the bubbles varied in size and were often too large to pass through the pulmonary capillaries. More importantly, injections of these types of ultrasound contrast agent can occur only near the region of interest because the microbubbles tend to go back into solution after a relatively short distance.

However, this approach is still being used, with the bubbles of gas being injected directly into vessels to enhance the reflectivity of the structures they perfuse. For instance, this approach has been used intraoperatively to better detect small hepatic carcinomas.[14] Carbon dioxide was mixed with physiologic saline and injected through a catheter positioned in the hepatic artery. Real-time ultrasound monitoring of the liver showed an immediate increase in the echogenicity of the liver parenchyma, which, after a few minutes, decreased at a faster rate than the tumor, allowing for its better visualization. Although there has been concern about the possibility of microbubbles of gas occluding capillaries in the brain or other organs, several reports have concluded that these agents are relatively safe.[15,16]

Researchers have continued to seek other methods of producing uniform small bubble sizes capable of passing through the capillary system and maintaining these over longer distances.[17,18] The most promising work in this area has consisted of microbubbles of gas incorporated within either a sugar matrix or human albumin.[19–21] Not only can these agents last for a much longer time, but their more uniform, smaller size allows them to pass through the capillaries. They remain intact long enough to be able to circulate at least once through the vascular system. In addition to ongoing research in the development of improved microbubble-containing ultrasound contrast agents, researchers have investigated other approaches, including the use of collagen spheres as well as solutions of various osmolarities.[22–25] In addition, perfluorochemicals also have been used as ultrasound contrast agents.[26]

In the development of ultrasound contrast agents, two approaches have been followed. In one, the agent increases the reflectivity of the blood or enhances the Doppler signals, or both[27,28]; in the other type, the agent is organ- or tumor-specific, because it tends to collect within or around abnormalities in such structures as the liver and spleen, increasing the difference in reflectivity (echogenicity) between the normal and adjacent abnormal tissue.[29]

Many approaches have been used, including the use of aqueous solutions, emulsions, suspensions, and encapsulated bubbles. Initial work in the area of aqueous solutions was performed by Ophir et al.,[22] who demonstrated that there was an increase in echogenicity within the kidney, both in vitro and in vivo, when contrast agents were injected intravascularly. Different solutions were tried, including sodium citrate and calcium disodium EDTA. However, the amount of solution needed to produce significant enhancement, as well as the concern over the toxicity of some of these solutions, has limited the usefulness of this approach.[30] Fink et al.[31] used emulsions of lipid in the hope that it would have the same effect as fatty infiltration of the liver by increasing the echogenicity of the tissue. It was found that the amount of lipid emulsion required to be injected to mimic fatty infiltration of the liver was prohibitively large.

The use of colloidal suspensions has shown some success in increasing the backscatter (echogenicity) of the tissue as well as enhancing the Doppler signal. Initial work by Ophir et al.[25] showed enhancement in canine livers in vivo using collagen microspheres 2.0 μm in diameter. It was hypothesized that the particles were picked up by the Kupffer cells of the liver. Mattrey et al.[32] used perfluoroctylbromide particles that were 0.5 μm in diameter. This agent produced an increased reflectivity in the liver and spleen, resulting in a rimlike region of increased echogenicity around tumors. Parker et al.[33] used iodipamide ethyl ester particles, 1 μm in size, to increase the backscatter within the rat liver. These small diameter particles permit intravenous injection followed by their rapid accumulation in the reticuloendothelial system in the liver and spleen. The contrast agent appears to be distributed throughout the normal liver rather than in tumors. Preliminary results suggest that the ultrasound attenuation can be controlled by the choice of the ultrasound frequency, particle concentration, and size.[33]

Of all the colloidal suspensions, the most promising, at the moment, appear to be perfluorochemicals (Imagent BP, Alliance Pharmaceuticals, San Diego, California), which are being tested to enhance the ultrasound backscatter in tissue and also the Doppler signals. In addition, this agent has shown some success in increasing the attenuation of tissue in computed tomography (CT).[29] Human experiments are ongoing in an attempt to demonstrate its effectiveness in different areas. Animal as well as human research has shown that it can enhance liver tumors after 24 to 48 hours and, more recently, that this contrast agent can enhance Doppler signals from the blood. Preliminary results also have shown that this agent increases the tissue reflectivity of the collecting system of rabbit kidneys.[34]

The reflectivity of perfluorocarbons is believed to be caused by their high density (1.9 g/ml) and low acoustic velocity (600 m/s), resulting in an acoustic impedance difference of 30 percent between the contrast agent and the adjacent tissues.[29] Because the impedance difference determines the strength of an echo, perfluorocarbons increase the echogenicity of the blood and tissues. The greater the amount given, the greater is the enhancement. For instance, using VX-2 tumors in rabbit kidneys, it has been shown that these hypovascular tumors appear to be less echogenic relative to the normal kidney after injection of this agent. In our own studies, the same effect has been seen in naturally occurring liver tumors in woodchucks, where the reflectivity of the normal tissue is increased relative to the less vascular tumors. A rim of increased reflectivity often appeared around the tumor (Fig. 3-2). The reverse can occur on occasion (i.e., a hyperechogenic liver tumor can appear to become isoechogenic after injection of perfluorochemicals). This is the "vanishing tumor effect" that has been reported in CT, where the difference between normal tissue and tumor is reduced after the injection of an iodinated contrast agent. It arises because the relative uptake of

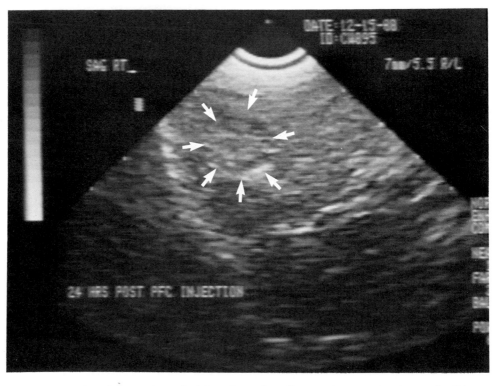

Fig. 3-2 Twenty-four hours after administration of perfluorocarbon, a rim (arrows) of increased reflectivity can be seen around a hepatoma in a woodchuck.

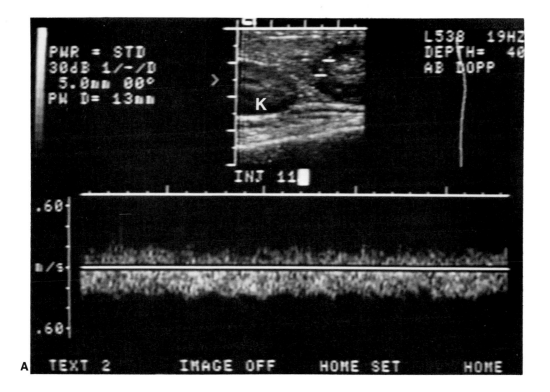

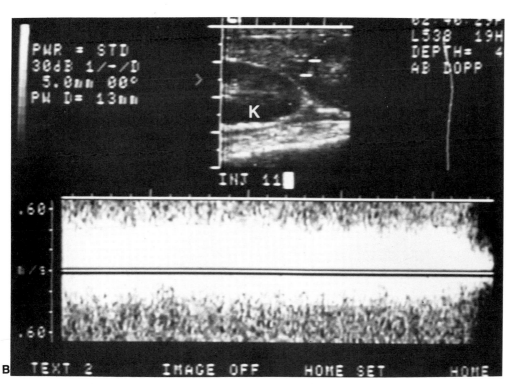

Fig. 3-3 Doppler spectrum signals obtained from edge of a hepatic tumor in a woodchuck **(A)** before and **(B)** after injection of air–filled albumin (Albunex). Note significant enhancement of spectral signals after intravenous contrast injection. K, kidney. (From Goldberg et al.,[28] with permission.)

the agent in the tissue is such that the attenuations of normal and abnormal tissues become equal. The effectiveness of this agent appears to be caused by its uptake by the reticuloendothelial system, with the effect increasing over several days. Perfluorochemicals also have been shown to enhance Doppler signals in both large and small blood vessels. The agent appears to be removed from the blood either by phagocytosis through the reticuloendothelial system or by evaporation through the lung over several days, or by both these mechanisms. Some adverse effects have been shown, including low back pain that was reversible when the infusion rate was reduced. Fever and trembling also have bee noted, regressing spontaneously over several hours.[29]

Many approaches have been tried in an attempt to encapsulate or trap gas bubbles. One of the first was the use of hydrogen gas trapped in gelatin capsules. The success of this approach was limited because of the 80-μm size of the particles. However, Carroll et al.[35] were able to show enhancement of tumor rims in rabbits with VX-2 tumors. Injections of this material had to be made directly into an artery perfusing the area of interest because the particles become trapped in the capillary system if injected peripherally.

Air-filled human albumin has been shown to traverse the pulmonary circulation, increasing the reflectivity of blood within the left atrium and ventricle. It has also been shown to pass through the capillary system, resulting in enhancement of the Doppler signals from various systemic arteries. These stable, air-filled human albumin microspheres (Albunex, Molecular Biosystems, San Diego, California) are from 1 to 8 μm (mean, 3.8 ± 2.5 μm) in diameter. The half-life of this contrast agent, when injected into blood, has been shown to be less than 1 minute. After

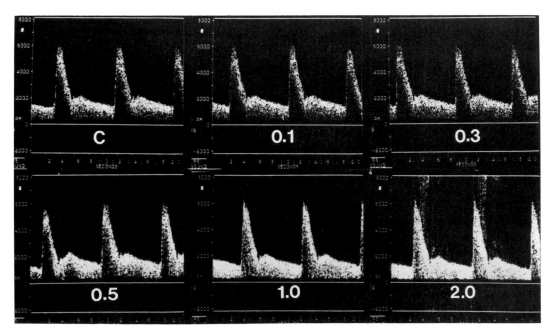

Fig. 3-4 Doppler spectrum measurements obtained from celiac artery with increasing intravenous doses (0.2 to 2.0 ml) of air-filled human albumin (Albunex) demonstrate progressive increase in signal intensity. C, control. (From Goldberg et al.,[28] with permission.)

3 minutes, more than 80 percent of the contrast agent was found in the liver. These microspheres are phagocytized by the reticuloendothelial system with byproducts returned to the blood and, within 24 hours, excreted in the urine.[36]

Recent investigations using naturally occurring hepatocellular tumors in woodchucks have shown that intravenous injections of Albunex produced immediate Doppler signal enhancement within the inferior vena cava, followed by enhancement within the abdominal aorta, hepatic artery, and its branches (Plate 3-1). Although the two-dimensional ultrasound images showed no perceivable change in tissue reflectivity of the normal parenchyma, tumor, or vessels, there was clear signal enhancement using Doppler (both spectral and color) (Fig. 3-3). This effect was found in both normal and tumor vessels. The greatest increase in Doppler intensity was apparent at the tumor periphery because the central portion tended to be less vascular and, in some cases, was even necrotic (Plate 3-2). As might be expected, the contrast agent effect increased in proportion to the dose (Fig. 3-4).[28]

STANDARDIZATION OF CONTRAST AGENTS

One of the problems with ultrasound contrast agents has been inadequate standardization in concentration, size, and stability. An attempt to solve these problems was the development of soluble saccharide (galactose) microparticles containing microbubbles of gas (Echovist, Schering, Berlin, Germany).[37] These microparticles have a medium diameter of 3.5 μm, with 99 percent being smaller than 12 μm. Trials have been carried out in both animals and humans in which contrast injected intravenously was imaged by ultrasound in the right atrium and ventricle. However, because the bubble sizes in suspension ranged from 5 to 15 μm, these mi-

croparticles could not pass easily from the right to the left side of the heart. Echovist, however, has been used for direct injection into arteries to visualize the organs the microparticles are perfusing.[38] For instance, when injected into flowing blood, the contrast agent could be visualized readily with both two-dimensional ultrasound imaging and Doppler (both spectral and color). When injected into the arterial supply of organs such as the kidney, this contrast material produced enhanced visualization of small vessels within the organ, producing a capillary blush seen on color Doppler as well as improving the signal-to-noise ratio of the Doppler signals obtained from vessels within this organ. Although this research was performed in animals, it shows promise for applications in humans. A limitation of this agent, however, is that it cannot be injected into a peripheral vein and still produce an effect in vessels and organs beyond the heart.

More recently, a new monosaccharide agent (Levovist, Schering, Berlin, Germany) has been produced to image the left side of the heart.[21,39] This agent is made from galactose but is produced with a slight change in its chemical composition to produce smaller, more stable, and uniform bubble sizes ranging from 2 to 8 μm in diameter, with 97 percent of the bubbles measuring less than 6 μm. This agent has been used successfully to visualize not only the right but also the left side of the heart. In addition, it is a nontoxic, neutral pH, biodegradable agent that is made from a naturally occurring substance. Levovist appears to be useful in delineating the circumference of the chambers of the heart as well as assisting in the calculation of ventricular ejection fraction and also should prove useful in visualizing and measuring left-to-right shunts. It has potential for producing myocardial enhancement, although more research is needed in this area.[39]

Because of its ability to traverse the cardiopulmonary circulation, we have evaluated

SHU 508 (Levovist) in noncardiac areas of the body. In animal studies, peripheral intravenous injections have resulted in enhancement of the Doppler signals (both spectral and color) in major vessels (both arteries and veins) throughout the body. Enhancement of smaller vessels in both liver and the kidneys has also been documented (Plate 3-3). Of more interest is its ability to enhance Doppler signals in the portal circulation, which means that the contrast agent has passed through two capillary beds. In addition, there is evidence of prolonged recirculation in excess of 3 minutes (Plate 3-4). Research with naturally occurring hepatocellular carcinomas in woodchucks has confirmed the ability of this contrast agent to increase the reflectivity of small vessels, not only within the normal portions of the liver but also within tumors (Plate 3-5). There was an increasing effect with increasing dose. The ultrasound contrast effects have also been shown in the celiac artery in doses as small as 0.025 ml/kg. Similar effects of the Doppler signal enhancement also have been shown in large animal models (dog and sheep). In the dog model, this agent produced enhancement of the Doppler signals in the vessels of the retina of the eye as well as the gallbladder, urinary bladder, and bowel walls. The lack of flow in an artificially produced region of renal ischemia was shown clearly (Plate 3-6).

NONVASCULAR DELIVERY OF CONTRAST AGENTS

Besides the use of ultrasound contrast agents through intra-arterial or intravenous injections, research has also shown the feasibility of using these agents to improve visualization of the endometrial cavity and Fallopian tube. Contrast agents have been introduced through catheters placed within the cervical os. Increased reflectivity (echogenicity) was seen within both the perfused Fallopian tube and the endometrial cavity.[40] However, initial results have shown no significant improvement over hysteroscopy or hysterosalpingography.[41] More work in this area will be needed before its efficacy can be established fully. An ultrasound contrast agent has also been placed within the urinary bladder in an attempt to visualize reflux into the ureters. Finally, injection through needles of a small amount of microbubble-containing material has been used to improve needle tip localization during ultrasound guided biopsy or drainage procedures.

ENHANCEMENT OF TUMOR DOPPLER SIGNALS

Abnormal blood flow associated with hepatocellular carcinomas, renal carcinomas, and breast tumors can be detected with the use of Doppler techniques.[42-44] With small malignant breast tumors, the low signal strength from moving scatterers (blood cells) is "diluted" by that of the adjacent stationary solid tissue, which is a limiting factor in the detection of these small tumors.[45] Ultrasound contrast agents should increase our ability to detect smaller vessels by enhancing backscatter in both tumor and normal vessels. The ability to detect the motion of blood in small vessels usually is limited in deep tissue. By increasing the reflectivity of the blood, an intravenously injected contrast agent enables better detection of blood flow in small, deep vessels than is possible with conventional Doppler techniques. For instance, signals enhanced by an ultrasound contrast agent were detected within woodchuck hepatocellular tumors from vessels that were not detected before the injection of the contrast agent. These experiments also suggest that an ultrasound contrast agent would help differentiate areas of normal vascularity from areas of reduced or absent flow caused by the presence of tumor necrosis. The demonstration of normal parenchymal arterial flow within areas that were considered abnormal may help distinguish tumors from pseudotumors, such as renal columns of Bertin. Ultrasound contrast agents also may aid in the detection of ischemia or occlusion. In cases of partial occlusion, the flow is often fast enough for normal Doppler detection. However, the quantity of blood that (with tissue attenuation) determines the signal strength passing through the narrowing may not be great enough to be detected with current Doppler equipment. Under certain circumstances, the introduction of more reflectors could aid in the delineation of the site of narrowing. Contrast agents also may aid in the visualization of collaterals caused by occlusion or severe stenosis. Although human studies are taking place using these gas-containing albumin or sugar-based particles to evaluate cardiac chambers and myocardial perfusion, other areas await Food and Drug Administration approval before further human research can commence in the United States.[21,36,39]

CONCLUSIONS

It is now clear that the most effective ultrasound contrast agent would be (1) nontoxic, (2) injectable intravenously, and (3) capable of passing through the pulmonary capillary and cardiac circulations to enhance detection of blood flowing in small vessels. Several potential ultrasound contrast agents have been or are now under development. Research in animals and limited results in humans suggest that ultrasound contrast agents will become commercially available in the not too distant future.

REFERENCES

1. Gramiak R, Shah PM: Echocardiography of the aortic root. Invest Radiol 3:356, 1968
2. Feigenbaum H, Stone J, Lee D et al: Identification of ultrasound echoes from the left ventricle by use of intracardiac injections of indocine green. Circulation 41:615, 1970
3. Kerber RE, Kioschos JM, Lauer RM: Use of an ultrasonic contrast method in the diagnosis of valvular regurgitation and intracardiac shunts. Am J Cardiol 34:722, 1974
4. Goldberg BB: Ultrasonic measurement of the aortic arch, right pulmonary artery, and left atrium. Radiology 101:383, 1971
5. Goldberg BB: Ultrasonic cholangiograpy, gray-scale B-scan evaluation of the common bile duct. Radiology 118:401, 1976
6. Ziskin MC, Bonakdapour A, Weinstein DP, Lynch PR: Contrast agents for diagnostic ultrasound. Invest Radiol 6:500, 1972
7. Feinstein SB, Ten Cate FJ, Zwehl W et al: Two-dimensional contrast echocardiography. I. In vitro development and quantitative analysis of echo contrast agents. J Am Coll Cardiol 3:14, 1984
8. Keller MW, Feinstein SB, Briller RA, Powsner SM: Automated production and analysis of echo contrast agents. J Ultrasound Med 5: 493, 1986
9. Reid CL, Kawanishi DT, McKay CR et al: Accuracy of evaluation of the presence and severity of aortic and mitral regurgitation by contrast 2-dimensional echocardiography Am J Cardiol 52:519, 1983
10. Sahn DJ, Valdez-Cruz LM: Ultrasonic contrast studies for the detection of cardiac shunts. J Am Coll Cardiol 3:978, 1984
11. Becher H, Schlief R, Lüderitz B: Improved sensitivity of color Doppler by SHU 454. Am J Cardiol 64:374, 1989
12. Tei C, Kondo S, Meerbaum S et al: Correlation of myocardial echo contrast disappearance rate ("washout") and severity of experimental coronary stenosis. J Am Coll Cardiol 3:39, 1984
13. Lang RM, Feinstein SB, Feldman T et al: Contrast echocardiography for evaluation of myocardial perfusion: effects of coronary angioplasty. J Am Coll Cardiol 8:232, 1986
14. Takada T, Yasuda H, Uchiyama K et al: Contrast-enhanced intraoperative ultrasonography of small hepatocellular carcinomas. Surgery 107:528, 1990
15. Bommer WJ, Shah P, Allen H et al: Contrast echocardiography. p. 1–10. Report of the American Society of Echocardiography, 1984
16. Gillam LD, Kaul S, Fallon JT et al: Functional and pathologic effects of multiple echocardiographic contrast injections on the myocardium, brain and kidney. J Am Coll Cardiol 3:687, 1984

17. Feinstein SB, Shah PM, Bing RJ et al: Microbubble dynamics visualized in the intact capillary circulation. J Am Coll Cardiol 3: 595, 1984

18. Reisner SA, Shapiro JR, Schwarz KQ, Meltzer RS: Sonication of echo-contrast agents: a standardized and reproducible method. J Cardiovasc Ultrason 7:273, 1988

19. Keller MN, Feinstein SB, Watson DD: Successful left ventricular opacification following peripheral venous injection of sonicated contrast agent: an experimental evaluation. Am Heart J 114:570, 1987

20. Berwing K, Schlepper M: Echocardiographic imaging of the left ventricle by peripheral intravenous injection of echocontrast agent. Am Heart J 115:399, 1988

21. Smith MD, Elion JL, McClure RR et al: Left heart opacification with peripheral venous injection of a new saccharide echo contrast agent in dogs. J Am Coll Cardiol 13:1622, 1989

22. Ophir J, McWhirt RE, Maklad NF: Aqueous solutions as potential ultrasonic contrast agents. Ultrason Imaging 1:265, 1979

23. Carroll BA, Turner R, Tichner G, Young SW: Microbubbles as ultrasonic contrast agents. Invest Radiol 14:374, 1979

24. Tyler TD, Ophir J, Maklad NF: In vivo enhancement of ultrasonic image luminance by aqueous solutions with high speed of sound. Ultrason Imaging 3:323, 1981

25. Ophir J, Gobuty A, McWhirt RE, Maklad NF: Ultrasonic backscatter from contrast producing collagen microspheres. Ultrason Imaging 2:67, 1980

26. Mattrey RF, Scheible FW, Gosink BB et al: Perfluorocytlbromide: a liver/spleen-specific and tumor-imaging ultrasound contrast material. Radiology 145:759, 1982

27. Hilpert PL, Mattrey RF, Mitten RM, Peterson T: IV injection of air-filled human albumin microspheres to enhance arterial Doppler signal: a preliminary study in rabbits. AJR 153:613, 1989

28. Goldberg B, Hilpert P, Burns P et al: Hepatic tumors: signal enhancement of Doppler US after intravenous injection of a contrast agent. Radiology 177:713, 1990

29. Mattrey RF: Perfluorooctylbromide: a new contrast agent for CT, sonography, and MR imaging. AJR 152:247, 1989

30. Ophir J, Parker KJ: Contrast agents in diagnostic ultrasound. Ultrasound Med Biol 15:319, 1989

31. Fink IJ, Miller DJ, Shawker TH: Lipid emulsions as contrast agents for hepatic sonography: an experimental study in rabbits. Ultrason Imaging 7:191, 1985

32. Mattrey RF, Strich G, Shelton RE et al: Perfluorochemicals as US contrast agents for tumor imaging and hepatosplenography: preliminary clinical results. Radiology 163:339, 1987

33. Parker KJ, Tuthill TA, Lerner RM, Violante MR: A particulate contrast agent with potential for ultrasound imaging of liver. Ultrasound Med Biol 13:555, 1987

34. Mattrey RF, Mitten R, Peterson T, Long CD: Vascular ultrasonic enhancement of tissues with perfluoroctylbromide for renal tumor detection. Radiology 165 (suppl):76, 1987

35. Carroll BA, Turner RJ, Tickner EG et al: Gelatin encapsulated nitrogen microbubbles as ultrasonic contrast agents. Invest Radiol 15: 260, 1980

36. Keller M, Glasheen W, Kaul S: Albunex: a safe and effective commercially produced agent for myocardial contrast echocardiography. J Am Soc Echocardiol 2:48, 198

37. Fritzsch TH, Schartl M, Siegert J: Preclinical and clinical results with an ultrasonic contrast agent. Invest Radiol 23 (suppl 1):S302, 1988

38. Mouaaouy AE, Becker HD, Schlief R et al: Rat liver model for testing intraoperative echo contrast sonography. Surg Endosc 4: 114, 1990

39. Schlief R, Staks T, Mahler M et al: Successful opacification of the left heart chambers on echocardiographic examination after intravenous injection of a new saccharide based contrast agent. Echocardiography 7:61, 1990

40. Deichert U, van de Sandt M, Lauth G, Daume E: Die Transvaginale hysterokontrastsonographie (HKSG). Geburtshilfe Frauenheilkd 48:835, 1988

41. Deichert U, Schlief R, van de Sandt M, Juhnke I: Transvaginal hysterosalpingo-contrast-sonography (Hy-Co-Sy) compared with conventional tubal diagnostics. Hum Reprod 4:418, 1989

42. Wells PNT, Halliwell M, Skidmore R et al: Tumour detection by ultrasonic Doppler blood-flow signals. Ultrasonics 15:231, 1977

43. Taylor KJW, Ramos I, Carter D et al: Correlation of Doppler US tumor signals with neovascular morphologic features. Radiology 166:57, 1988

44. Ramos I, Taylor KJW, Kier R et al: Tumor vascular signals in renal masses: detection with Doppler US. Radiology 168:633, 1988

45. Burns PN, Halliwell M, Wells PNT, Webb AJ: Ultrasonic Doppler studies of the breast. Ultrasound Med Biol 8:127, 1982

4

Advances in Imaging Techniques

Peter N. T. Wells

TRANSDUCERS

Arguably, the transducer is the main component in any ultrasound imaging system. It converts electrical signals into ultrasound and controls the beam and pulse shapes, and it produces electrical signals in response to echoes received from within the patient. The ideal transducer is efficient as a transmitter, is sensitive as a receiver, has good pulse characteristics with very low-amplitude ringing, and has a wide angle response when used in a focused or steered array.

Transducer Materials

Ferroelectric ceramics are nowadays almost universally used as medical diagnostic ultrasound transducers.[1] The reason for this is that ceramic materials have very high piezoelectric and mechanical coupling coefficients. This means that they are efficient transmitters and sensitive receivers. Unfortunately, however, ceramics have characteristic acoustic impedances that are very much greater than those of water and soft tissues. Consequently, well-designed impedance

matching layers are necessary to provide efficient broadband operation.[2] Various types of ultrasound transducers are in routine clinical use; they include single-element disks (often concave to focus the ultrasound beam and sometimes fitted with plastic lenses) and annular and linear arrays. The linear arrays may be up to about 10 cm long, with up to about 300 elements; these long arrays may be flat or convex, the latter producing a kind of sector scan. When used with modern scanners, linear and convex arrays often have electronically controlled focusing at a suitable fixed depth on transmission, with dynamically swept focusing on reception.[3] Sometimes, linear array transducers are used for color-flow imaging (see Ch. 8); to obtain a suitable Doppler angle, the beam may then be steered into a trapezoidal format, or a wedge may be used, when examining vessels running roughly parallel to the skin surface. Shorter versions of linear arrays, typically about 10 mm long with up to about 100 elements, are operated as phase arrays to produce sector scans.[4]

Recently, there has been considerable interest

in the possibility of using piezoelectric plastic transducers in medical ultrasound diagnosis. Polyvinylidene difluoride and its derivatives[5] have much lower characteristic acoustic impedances than the ceramics and so provide a much better match with water and soft tissues, thus eliminating the need for impedance matching layers. Plastic transducers are also relatively free from multiple mode resonances (in comparison with the ceramics), and this is an important advantage, particularly when operating off-axis in an array. The main disadvantage of plastic transducers is that they have relatively low dielectric constants, requiring high driving voltages and giving poor noise performances.

At present, the most promising new transducer materials are the piezoelectric composites. These consist of plastic polymer substrates within which small particles (or, ideally, rods) of piezoelectric ceramic are embedded. They combine characteristic acoustic impedance approaching that of purely plastic materials with the high efficiency and sensitivity and the low electrical impedance of the ceramics,[6] and they are relatively free from lateral resonance effects.[7]

Piezoelectric composites are now beginning to be used in commercially available probes. It is their broadband capability that is perceived to be their principal advantage. Transducer manufacturers, however, are likely to be motivated by the facility with which curved transducers can be constructed with these materials and because the expense of producing some types of specialized probes may bring them (just) into the range of high-cost disposables.

Besides probes for transcutaneous and intracavitary (i.e., intraesophageal, intrarectal, and intravaginal) applications, devices are available for scanning from the lumens of blood vessels (see Ch. 2). These miniature catheter-mounted transducers may be mechanically driven, or the beam steering may be achieved by means of arrays[8]; generally, a radial scanning pattern is used. The probes usually operate at frequencies of up to about 20 MHz; penetrations of about a centimeter are typical, and the images have a resolution (close to the probe) of about a tenth of a millimeter.

Implications for System Performance

The improved pulse response of modern ultrasound transducers, and particularly the low amplitude of the ringing and other noise-producing phenomena, means that the dynamic range of the imaging systems can be increased. The principal advantage of this is improvement in contrast resolution. Thus, for example, anechoic cysts appear as more nearly clear black areas in the image and the subtle gray-level differences of normal liver tissue texture and hepatic metastases can be more obvious.

Modern ultrasound transducers also have wideband capability. This means that the frequency can be changed, at least over a limited range, without the need to change the probe. Typically, a 7.5-MHz probe can operate satisfactorily at any frequency in the 5- to 10-MHz band. Although the attenuation in tissue determines the maximum usable frequency at the maximum depth of penetration, there is no fundamental reason why the resolution over the whole image should have to be uniform. Indeed, it is not. It is pointed out in Chapter 9 that the frequency can be swept downward with time in the same way that swept gain is applied to compensate for attenuation.[9] The imaging system can be considered to have two bandwidth-limiting components. The first of these components is the tissue; because attenuation in tissue increases with frequency, the tissue behaves like a low-pass filter. The second bandwidth-limiting component is the transducer, and modern transducers have bandwidths approaching 100 percent of their center frequencies.

There is a debate about whether it is better to sweep the frequency to which the receiver is tuned continuously with time to optimize the resolution over the entire image, or to select the frequency to provide optimum resolution at the particular depth of interest in the study that is actually being performed. From the point of view of the person performing the scan and viewing the image, continuously swept frequency is likely to be better because it does not require any operator intervention and it increases the chance of noticing details of significance in unexpected parts of the image. However, selection of the optimum frequency for the depth of interest minimizes the possibility of hazard to the overlying structures, because higher-frequency components in the pulse, which would be lost by attenuation in the overlying tissues without providing any useful information, simply are not transmitted at all. In many clinical situations, this is probably an academic argument, but it could have practical relevance in, for example, obstetrics and ophthalmology.

IMAGING SYSTEM HARDWARE

Aperture Optimization

It has already been pointed out that tissue inhomogeneity limits the improvement in resolution that can be obtained by increasing the aperture of a focused ultrasound transducer. The size of the aperture in relation to the wavelength also controls the relative amplitudes of the main lobe of the ultrasound beam and its side lobes. This can easily be understood by considering what happens to the beam as the aperture is increased in size. When the aperture is very small, ultrasound is radiated equally in all directions: the transducer is said to be a "point source." As the

aperture is increased, however, the beam becomes more concentrated in the forward direction; in the case of a disk transducer, the beam is symmetric about its central axis normal to the surface of the source. At the same time, however, the beam begins to develop side lobes that consist of coaxial conically shaped regions surrounding the main beam. Moreover, the relative amplitudes of these side lobes also increase.

So far, we have considered how to optimize the choice of frequency to achieve the best imaging performance. Although the aperture of the transducer cannot be adjusted dynamically to control the shape of the transmitted beam, it can be changed during reception.[10] Moreover, by using different sizes of aperture on transmit and receive, it is possible to place the minima of one beam near the side-lobe maxima of others, thus achieving side-lobe suppression.[11] If patients consisted of homogeneous tissue, it would be possible to select the optimum aperture for imaging at any chosen depth. It is well known, however, that the images of some patients are obviously of high quality, whereas other patients are difficult to image satisfactorily. Better results may be obtained with the latter group of patients by reducing the size of the aperture of the transducer. In any event, it is usually best to arrange for the size of the receiving aperture to increase dynamically with depth, thus maintaining a roughly constant f-number (equal to the ratio of the focal length to the size of the aperture).[12]

Analog or Digital Circuit Operation

Until recently, ultrasound imaging instruments used entirely analog circuits. An analog circuit is one in which the output signals are derived directly from the input signals; frequency selection (tuning), amplification (which may have a linear or nonlinear transfer characteristic), demodulation (detection or rectification), and signal processing (e.g., differentiation for edge detection) are typical of the operations that may be performed. The development of relatively inexpensive digital circuit components, however, has made it feasible for equipment designers to begin to adopt digital techniques in ultrasound scanners.

Digital techniques were first used to control the function of the scanner and to provide alphanumeric information in the display. Then followed some signal processing features, such as the frequency analysis of Doppler signals by fast Fourier transform. Most recently, it has become practicable to digitize the ultrasound signals before demodulation. For satisfactory results, digitization at three to five times the maximum ultrasound frequency is necessary, so sampling rates of 20 MHz are typical. These high speeds are necessary because delay quantization errors can cause increased side lobe amplitudes, thereby limiting the dynamic range.[13] The dynamic range needs to be at least 30 dB after swept gain control (corresponding to 5-bit quantization). Twelve-bit quantization is just within the realm of possibility at 20-MHz sampling frequency; this corresponds to a dynamic range of 72 dB. Without swept gain, the dynamic range required for satisfactory performance is at least 100 dB; consequently, some degree of dynamic range compression is currently necessary if digitization is to be performed in advance of the swept gain control circuit. If a transducer array is being used for beam forming or steering, or both, current economics require that swept gain is applied in the signal path of each receiving transducer element before digitization.

In principle, digital operation leads to flexible control of an imaging system. Starting at the front end of the system, where it is attached to the transducer, beam forming, steering, and aperture control can be chosen by software as can the ultrasound receiving frequency passband. The beam forming and steering functions are particularly important, because the digital techniques replace analog circuits that have to be switched or voltage controlled and that are prone to drift with time and changing temperature. The precision with which the time delays can be selected has much to do with the geometry of the ultrasound beam, including the extent of the artifact-producing side lobes. As the ultrasound signal moves farther from the front end and toward the display, the demands on digital processing circuits become progressively less severe. Nowadays, demodulation, video amplification, and pre- and postprocessing functions economically can be fully digital. Besides traditional swept gain, which controls the sensitivity of the receiver according to depth, it is easy to provide adjustment of swept gain across the scan plane; this can be especially helpful when structure boundaries to be studied. Moreover, the cost of image storage is inexpensive, so it is easy to include features such as ciné-loop replay and frame averaging. Moreover, combining gray-scale and color images in a single display is commonplace.

To make use of regular video circuit components, such as television displays, frame stores, and video tape recorders, it is necessary to convert the image as it is obtained in the format of the scan to a television raster signal. Typically, the format of the scan is a sector, a trapezium, or a circular segment. Nowadays, a digital scan converter is used for this task. The process maps the scan data (often in polar coordinates) to Cartesian coordinates. The resulting image is characterized by fringe artifacts, oversampling, missing pixels, and blocks.[14] Without further processing, such an image would be unacceptable by modern standards. The simplest method of improving the image is by nearest neighbor interpolation, which maps the sampled data to the nearest pixel in the digital scan converter. Unfortunately, the result of this approach depends on whether many scan lines pass through individual pixels (as is the case close to a sector scanning transducer) or many blank pixels occur between sparse lines (as at the deeper parts of a sector scan). Although it is easy to remove the fringes, the location errors remain. One solution to this problem is by the "uniform ladder algorithm," in which the memory is in the form of a rectangle (instead of a sector). This is achieved by controlling the sampling rate across the sector according to the horizontal depth from the center of the sector, rather than sampling at constant rate.[15] Is it then only necessary to fill the gaps between the pixels in the horizontal direction.

TISSUE CHARACTERIZATION

For years, scientists have been seeking clues in ultrasound signals that could lead to the identification of the histologic and pathologic characteristics of the examined tissues.[16] Radiologists often can identify pathology by image inspection, especially when there are only a few feasible alternatives. For example, it may be possible to distinguish between cystic and solid lesions because of the relatively low attenuation and echogenicity of the liquid contents of cysts. Practical problems exist, however, in distinguishing between the histologies of solid lesions and, in particular, in characterizing benign and malignant tumors.

In principle, at least seven different physical properties of tissues can be observed by ultrasound.

Attenuation of Ultrasound. Attenuation can be measured either by through transmission (either linearly[17] or by computed tomography[18]), by the decrement of echo amplitude with increasing range,[19] or by the downward shift in the frequency of echo signals.[20] The situation is complicated further because the inhomogeneities in some tissues (such as skeletal muscle) are aligned directionally and attenuation consequently may be anisotropic.

Speed of Ultrasound. The speed of ultrasound (which, like attenuation, may be anisotropic) can be measured by through transmission[16,17] or by triangulation.[21]

Characteristic Acoustic Impedance. The characteristic acoustic impedance of a material is equal to the product of its density and the speed of ultrasound within it. It can be estimated by correcting echo amplitude measurements from boundaries between tissues for their geometries and for attenuation and beam diffraction effects.[22]

Scattering of Ultrasound. The scattering characteristics of tissues can be specified in terms of angular and frequency dependencies and time variation.[23]

Nonlinear Propagation. The nonlinearity of signal propagation can be measured as a function of ultrasound intensity.[24]

Tissue Elasticity. The elasticity of tissue can be related to motion detected as the result of physiologic or applied forces.[25]

Blood Flow. The volume rate and pulsatility of blood flow is related to the properties of associated tissues. It can be detected and measured by techniques based on the Doppler effect.[26]

Despite all this effort, much of which was expended some time ago, it is only through image inspection and Doppler studies that tissue characterization has achieved routine clinical application.[27] Different tissues generally do not have sufficiently different attenuations, speeds, or even recognizable scattering characteristics to be distinguishable by ultrasound in practically relevant ways. Not enough is known about acoustic impedance and nonlinearity, which are in any case difficult to measure accurately, to say whether they could be useful. The prospects are not encouraging. Finally, motion studies, which are in their infancy, can be applied only in a few well-defined situations, although it could be speculated that they might be particularly relevant to the thyroid, breast, and prostate.

For the future, it might be argued that the best prospect for progress in ultrasound tissue characterization is through the development of ultrasound contrast agents, which are discussed in some detail in Chapter 3. If contrast agent systems and targeting schemes could be developed to solve the problems of sensitivity, selectivity, and toxicity, ultrasound might be able to take over many of the roles of nuclear medicine inexpensively and safely. They would avoid the use of ionizing radiation, and they might be safer, cheaper, and more useful.

ADVANCES IN DOPPLER

Doppler was first used in clinical diagnosis more than 30 years ago. Although the pioneers were interested in cardiac function, it was for the measurement of fetal heart rate as an aid in better obstetric care that the method was popularized. Then, continuous-wave Doppler techniques were applied to the investigation of peripheral and cerebral arterial disease. In the 1970s, the duplex scanner was invented, and pulsed Doppler techniques were shown to be enormously useful in cardiology, as well as for the study of localized vascular disease and for physiologic investigations.

During the past 5 years, advances in color-flow imaging (see Ch. 8) and blood flow measurement have been dramatic. The established method of blood flow volume rate measurement is dealt with in Chapter 10. Here, it is worth drawing attention to yet another novel approach to solving this problem.[28] It is, in effect, a real-time ultrasound Doppler C-scan system. A small two-di-

mensional transducer array is used to provide uniform insonation of a plane at some chosen depth along the ultrasound beam. The blood vessel in which it is desired to measure the blood flow is arranged to pass through the uniformly insonated plane; although the angles are not critical, it is best to ensure that the flow direction is as near to normal as possible to the insonated plane. Because the transducer is a two-dimensional array, it is possible to have a mutiplicity of separate receiving channels operating simultaneously, each channel being associated with its own highly focused receiving beam. The receiving beams are steered individually so that the entire plane of insonation is examined simultaneously at many points in real-time. Consequently, the instrument derives an instantaneous map of the flow profile through the plane. The instantaneous volume under the flow profile is equal to the blood volume flow rate independent of the Doppler angle and tissue attenuation and (at least, to a first approximation) inhomogeneity in the overlying tissues.

CONCLUSION

Ultrasound diagnosis is a mature technology in that it has an established and vitally important role in modern imaging practice. The advances that have taken place in the past few years have led to startling improvements in system performance and image quality. Moreover, the opportunities for further innovation seem never to have been brighter or more promising than they are at this moment. Dramatic progress can confidently be predicted for the next decade, especially in transducer materials and construction, signal processing, and image management and display.

REFERENCES

1. Hunt JW, Arditi M, Foster FS: Ultrasound transducers for pulse-echo medical imaging. IEEE Trans Biomed Eng 30:453, 1983

2. Inoue T, Ohta M, Takahashi S: Design of ultrasonic transducers with multiple acoustic matching layers for medical application. IEEE Trans Ultrason Ferroelect Freq Contr 34:8, 1987

3. Wells PNT: Physics and instrumentation. p. 1. In Goldberg BB, Wells PNT (eds): Ultrasonics in Clinical Diagnosis. Churchill Livingstone, Edinburgh, 1983

4. von Ramm OT, Smith SW: Beam steering with linear arrays. IEEE Trans Biomed Eng 30:438, 1983

5. Kimura K, Hashimoto N, Ohigashi H: Performance of a linear array transducer of vinylidene fluoride trifluoroethylene copolymer. IEEE Trans Sonics Ultrason 32:566, 1985

6. Gururaja TR, Schulze WA, Cross LE, Newnham RE: Piezoelectric composite materials for ultrasonic transducer applications. Part II: Evaluation of ultrasonic medical applications. IEEE Trans Sonics Ultrason 32:499, 1985

7. Richter KP, Reibold R, Molkenstruck W: Sound field characteristics of composite pulse transducers. Ultrasonics 29:76, 1991

8. Gussenhoven WJ, Bom N, Roelandt J: Intravascular Ultrasound 1991. Kluwer, Dordrecht, 1991

9. Claesson I, Salomonsson G: Frequency- and depth-dependent compensation of ultrasonic signals. IEEE Trans Ultrason Ferroelect Freq Contr 35:582, 1988

10. Maslak SH: Computed sonography. p. 1. In Sanders RC, Hill MC (eds). Ultrasonic Annual 1985. Raven Press, New York, 1985

11. Moshfeghi M: Side-lobe suppression for ultrasonic imaging arrays. Ultrasonics 17:322, 1987

12. Dietz DI, Parks SI, Linzer M: Expanding-aperture annular array. Ultrason Imaging 1:56, 1979

13. Magnin PG, von Ramm OT, Thurstone FL: Delay quantization error in phased array images. IEEE Trans Sonics Ultrason 28:305, 1981

14. Maginness MG: Signal processing, image storage, and display. p. 40. In Wells PNT, Ziskin MC (eds): New Techniques and Instrumentation in Ultrasonography. Churchill Livingstone, New York, 1980

15. Lee MH, Kim JH, Park SB: Analysis of scan conversion algorithm for a real-time sector scanner. IEEE Trans Med Imaging 5:96, 1986

16. Greenleaf JF: Tissue Characterization with Ultrasound. Vols. I and II. CRC Press, Boca Raton, Florida, 1986

17. Wells PNT: Biomedical Ultrasonics. Academic Press, London, 1977

18. Greenleaf JF, Kenue SK, Rajagopalan B et al: Breast imaging by ultrasonic computer-assisted tomography. p. 599. In Metherell AF (ed): Acoustic Imaging. Vol. 8. Plenum Press, New York, 1980

19. Mountford RA, Wells PNT: Ultrasonic liver scanning: the quantitative analysis of the normal A-scan. Phys Med Biol 17:14, 1972

20. Kuc R, Schwartz M: Estimating the acoustic attenuation coefficient slope for liver from reflected ultrasound signals. IEEE Trans Sonics Ultrason 26:353, 1979

21. Robinson DE, Chan F, Wilson LW: Measurement of velocity of propagation from ultrasonic pulse-echo data. Ultrasound Med Biol 8:413, 1982

22. Herment A, Perroneau P, Vayse M: A new method of obtaining acoustic impedance profile for characterization of tissue structures. Ultrasound Med Biol 5:321, 1979

23. Dickinson RJ: Reflection and scattering. p. 225. In Hill CR (ed): Physical Principles of Medical Ultrasonics. Ellis Horwood, Chichester, 1986

24. Law WK, Frizzell LA, Dunn F: Determination of the nonlinearity parameter B/A of biological media. Ultrasound Med Biol 11:307, 1985

25. Tristam M, Barbosa DC, Cosgrove DO et al: Ultrasonic studies of in vivo kinetic characteristics of human tissues. Ultrasound Med Biol 12:927, 1986

26. Burns PN, Halliwell M, Wells PNT, Webb AJ: Ultrasonic Doppler studies of the breast. Ultrasound Med Biol 8:127, 1982

27. Taylor KJW, Wells PNT: Tissue characterization. Ultrasound Med Biol 15:421, 1989

28. Moser U, Anliker M, Schumacher P: Ultrasonic synthetic aperture imaging to measure 2D velocity fields in real time. IEEE Int Symp Circuits Syst 1:738, 1991

5
Speckle Reduction

Jeffrey C. Bamber

Despite the high level of sophistication now achieved in ultrasound imaging instrumentation, the images still look different from and, to some eyes, inferior to those generated by many other medical imaging modalities. As a result of the dominating effect of coherent speckle noise, the images have a characteristic mottled or granular structure, which causes many anatomic features to break up and meaningless fine detail to appear where there should only be a uniform gray level.

The best achievable (diffraction limited) resolution of an ultrasound scanner is commonly measured by judging some level of point spatial discrimination, such as the closest separation that can be achieved for two wire targets in water while their images can still be distinguished (see Ch. 9). The size that an object needs to be before it is visually distinguishable from its background, however, is a function of both spatial and contrast resolution. Contrast discrimination in B-scan imaging is determined by the acoustic backscattering contrast between tissue regions, signal processing in the scanner and display (including viewing conditions), and any noise that may be present. Electronic noise, which adds to the echo signal, limits penetration depth, but the speckle noise, a multiplicative modulation of the echo signal, usually limits the contrast resolution. As a consequence, the diffraction limited spatial resolution rarely is achieved for most practical objects.

The spatial frequency spectrum of speckle noise is (1) almost identical in form to and is superimposed on the imaging system modulation transfer function (MTF), and (2) the MTF of the human visual system indicates a pronounced maximum sensitivity to structure with a spatial frequency in the region of one to three cycles per degree.[1] The former was said to be a "worst possible result" because it minimizes diagnostic information transfer. The spatial frequency stated in the latter is close to the spatial frequency for speckle displayed on ultrasound scanners at typical viewing distances and therefore is likely to attract a viewer's attention at the expense of diagnostically important information. Speckle may have a further distracting effect in real-time scanning if the speckle noise fluctuation rate happens to lie close to the frequency of visual peak temporal contrast sensitivity.[1] It certainly has been shown that the presence of speckle in an image reduces the temporal contrast sensitivity of human vision.[2] This may reduce the likelihood of observers being able to use motion information to detect otherwise noise-limited signals (e.g., arterial walls).[1] It has also been shown[3] that both low-contrast lesions (Fig. 5-1) and semiperiodic textures[4] are difficult to detect in the presence of speckle.

For more than a decade, a search has been underway to demonstrate a successful and practical method of improving the contrast resolution in ultrasound B-scans by removing the speckle without cost to other factors of image quality. As we shall see later, this has been neither straightforward nor entirely successful, but good progress has been made and the rewards for success might be considerable. In general, it seems reasonable to expect that if speckle were not present in ultrasound images, it would be easier to perceive (1) small differences in mean image brightness, (2) small high-contrast targets, (3) low-contrast objects, and (4) changes in the nonspeckle component of image texture. Speckle also adds an undesirable statistical fluctuation to any quantities extracted from the image.

Speckle in real-time ultrasound scans also may carry useful information, particularly about the motion of unresolved structure, but such additional information is probably best extracted by digital processing and encoded using (for example) color.[5,6]

ORIGIN AND BEHAVIOR OF SPECKLE

Speckle is the term used to describe the fluctuations in signal level caused by interference between waves received simultaneously apparently originating from the same point in the object. The apparent echo level can vary rapidly from nothing, in the case of complete destructive interference, to a high value when all components add up constructively. The phenomenon is common to all imaging modalities based on coherent forms of radiation, including optical and radar systems[7]—viewing the human body with coherent sound is rather like trying to picture our normal world under the constraints of the scintillating, shimmering effect of laser light. There are several possible mechanisms for the production of speckle noise in ultrasound systems. In the "rough volume" model,[8–11] a region of the object (known as the resolution cell of the imaging system)

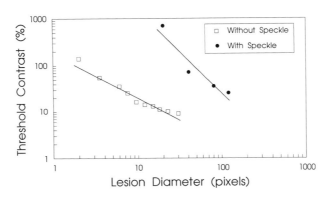

Fig. 5-1 Experimentally determined contrast thresholds for visual detection of uniform disks against uniform backgrounds (□□□) and speckle modulated disks against speckle modulated backgrounds (●●●) (speckle cell ≈ 3.5 axial by 9 lateral pixels). Note, for example, that a speckle-free "lesion" of 50 percent higher luminance than its background was visible at about one-eighth the diameter necessary to see it in speckle. (Adapted from Lowe et al.,[3] with permission.)

that corresponds to a point in the image is said to contain scattering structure too fine to be resolved (i.e., there are many sources of scattered waves within the resolution cell). This case represents the volume analog of the case of laser speckle produced by coherent light scattering from a rough surface.[12] The simultaneous arrival or integration of signals also can be the result of multiple scattering, high side or grating lobe levels, and any factors (e.g., an inhomogeneous propagation medium) that distort the phase of the received wave across the receiving aperture. The last of these applies because acoustic receivers are phase-sensitive.

The detailed image structure in regions of full speckle bears no obvious relationship to the tissue structure (i.e., positions of the scatterers), which would simply be smoothed by an incoherent imaging. The general properties of the chaotic pattern (or texture) of speckle may be described by statistical methods, although the detail itself is determined entirely by the physical scattering process (i.e., it is deterministic): if nothing moves or changes, the speckle pattern is completely repeatable. Fully developed speckle, predicted by the rough volume model when more than about eight scatterers are randomly distributed within the resolution cell, has predictable global properties.[13–16] When not corrupted by nonlinear signal processing, the shape of its gray-level probability density function (PDF) is a Rayleigh distribution with a mean value equal to about 1.92 times the standard deviation (this ratio is known as the *signal-to-noise ratio* [SNR]), and a typical speckle cell has a size and shape that are about the same size and shape as the resolution cell. The speckle cell size varies within the image because of the diffraction field of the transducer and the presence of frequency-dependent attenuation. Furthermore, when there is multiple scattering, phase cancellation in the transducer or side/grating lobe interference mechanisms are dominant, and a finer speckle pattern results, the cell size of which

tends not to be representative of the main resolution cell.

If the object contains some (even incompletely) resolved structure or some underlying regular distribution of scatterers, the properties of the image texture change, so that they are no longer entirely characteristic of the imaging system but may be used to classify the structure of the object.[14–20] A single measure such as the SNR may, however, be inadequate because changes in SNR may occur, caused by either changes in scatterer number density or their distribution, both of which represent structural departures from the situation of fully developed speckle.[16,21]

SPECKLE REDUCTION METHODS

The local pattern of speckle only changes (or decorrelates) if a different part of the object is imaged, the scattering structure is viewed from a different angle, or a different combination of acoustic wavelengths is used in forming the image. Most speckle reduction methods rely on varying one or more of these parameters to generate multiple images with uncorrelated speckle patterns, which are then averaged to reduce the contrast of the speckle modulation. In synthetic aperture radar (SAR) imagery, this is known as diversity or multilook processing. For electromagnetic radiation, speckle also decorrelates with changing polarization,[22] and the method of "polarization diversity" is very effective in suppressing SAR speckle[23] (an option not available with longitudinal acoustic waves). In medical ultrasound imaging, the process of averaging many images is known as compounding. It is only fully effective if images with uncorrelated speckle patterns can be generated, in which case the improvement in SNR is in proportion to the square root of the number of images. Unfortunately, this process always results in some loss of spatial resolution. It is possible, however, to achieve a compromise between loss of spatial resolution and gain in contrast resolution by averaging a number of partially decorrelated speckle patterns.[24]

As illustrated by Figure 5-1, spatial and contrast resolution are linked inextricably. Improvement in spatial resolution (by increasing the bandwidth or aperture) results in a lower-contrast threshold for lesion visibility without changing the speckle SNR, because more speckle cells per unit area are available to sample the scattering level within the lesion.[25] Speckle modulation severely distorts the signal PDF, positively skewing it so that the most frequently occurring values are relatively decreased. For the display of optical images degraded by speckle noise, a gray-scale logarithmic transform has been applied to correct for this distortion.[26] This is not strictly speckle reduction, but a similar display transform is, for other reasons, applied as a routine part of gray-scale ultrasound signal processing.

Spatial and Temporal Compounding (Including Linear Filtering)

Spatial averaging has been applied over images obtained by translating the scan plane,[27] and may be a good technique for anatomic structures that vary more slowly in the direction across the scan plane (e.g., perhaps in the neck, limbs). Spatial averaging of this kind is also the basis for the display of three-dimensional data sets by means of the "summed voxel projection" rendering method.[28,29] Such displays are, to a large extent, free of speckle. Averaging over several frames obtained from a real-time scanner[30,31] is entirely equivalent to spatial compounding but involves less control over which frames are averaged. It is unlikely that small physiologic movements produce different speckle patterns but with essentially identical anatomic information,[32,33] because the motion needed to produce speckle decorrelation is a

distance equal to the displayed size of the smallest structures resolved. Sufficient temporal compounding to reduce the SNR always results in blurring of resolved structure (Fig. 5-2). For real-time imaging, frame rate is also sacrificed, and because of the deterministic nature of the speckle noise, the speckle reappears whenever the transducer or the object, or both, stops moving. Speckle smoothing caused by the time integrating effect of human vision[33] occurs, if at all, only at very low light levels after dark adaptation.[1]

Despite its inherent limitations and disadvantages, the technique of temporal compounding is simple to implement in real-time and is sufficiently successful that many manufacturers have incorporated it in their equipment in the form of a variable "persistence" or "temporal processing" control. To the author's knowledge, however, no study has yet been undertaken to discover whether this form of processing has had an impact on diagnostic accuracy. The author's experience is that when imaging stationary organs, medical personnel often prefer some moderate amount of frame averaging and that they learn to control the degree of image blurring in a dynamic and interactive manner by varying the speed at which the transducer is moved through the volume of interest. Notwithstanding fundamental arguments about the undesirability of displaying speckle in ultrasound images, these practical observations of the way an existing (imperfect) speckle reduction method is used are encouraging and suggest that any method that could reduce speckle without suffering from other penalties (e.g., loss of resolution or frame rate) would be welcomed by many practicing ultrasonologists.

Image filtering often is discussed separately from compounding, but linear filtering (i.e., smoothing) is nothing more than spatial averaging (compounding) within a single image. It reduces speckle but results in blur-

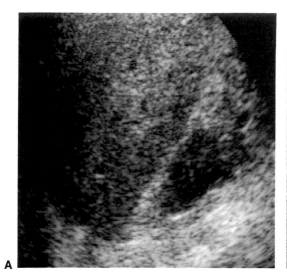 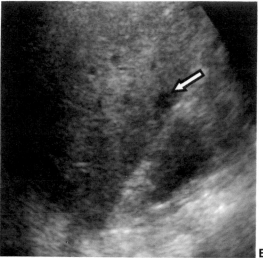

A B

Fig. 5-2 Spatial compounding obtained by using temporal averaging in combination with object/transducer motion. **(A)** Single frame from real-time sector scan of liver. **(B)** Spatially compounded version showing enhanced visibility of a suspected lesion (arrow), obtained by keeping the transducer in motion while averaging six sequential frames.

ring of resolved structures and meaningful texture.[26,34] Even when the filter is controlled carefully so that its spatial frequency cut-off is tailored to the resolution limit of the system,[35] relatively little improvement appears to be obtained. However, many real-time ultrasound scanners incorporate edge enhancement. This tends to emphasize the speckle pattern but, in so doing, may enhance the perception of moving unresolved tissue structure.

Angle Compounding

It is possible to decorrelate speckle without imaging a different part of the object by changing the angle of incidence of the sound beam on the structure to be visualized.[36–40] This method represents one of the more successful forms of compounding and often has the additional desirable effect of enhancing the visibility of large-scale (nearly specularly reflecting) anatomic boundaries.[41] Application is limited to regions accessible through a large acoustic window, but when access is

available over 360 degrees, virtually speckle-free imaging with visually striking contrast resolution is possible,[42,43] which in the examples cited takes the form of breast architecture delineated with surprising clarity. Degradation of point resolution, caused by differences in acoustical path length and refraction, and loss of other diagnostically useful information, such as shadowing or enhancement behind regions of varying attenuation coefficient, resulted (when compound scanners were available) in the practice of performing breast examinations using both simple and compound B-scans.[36] Tissue movement is also currently a limitation, but this is likely to be less of a problem when parallel processing in the receiver is used to increase frame rate.[44]

All approaches to angle compounding have one thing in common: the available acoustic aperture (i.e., the angle or solid angle of acoustic access) is divided into subapertures, so that a set of detected images may be formed by coherently focusing within each subaperture and the final image is obtained incoherently by averaging the image set. Several novel approaches to speckle reduction through aperture subdivision have been published, including the division of a conical ("axicon") transducer into sectors[45] and the division of a circular transducer into a "Maltese cross" configuration.[46] A method related to aperture subdivision is that of controlling the spatial coherence of the ultrasound beam using a random phase screen.[47] The cost of speckle reduction by aperture subdivision is a loss of point target resolution, because the lateral beamwidth of the incoherent imaging system becomes that of the reduced aperture size. Despite this trade-off in determinants of image quality, there is a worthwhile benefit to low-contrast lesion detectability for aperture subdivision ratios up to about 3:1 or 4:1.[38,39]

Frequency Compounding

Averaging over images made at different frequencies, whether using filtering methods, frequency modulated pulses, or phase modulated pulses,[38,48–54] is potentially fast, it permits a narrow access window to be used, and there is no need to rely on multiple propagation paths being equal or to lose the diagnostic signs because of shadowing and enhancement. This is not thought, however, to be a successful approach. The bandwidth of an ultrasound transducer and the frequency dependence of ultrasound attenuation in tissues make it difficult to achieve statistically independent speckle images without loss of resolution. Subdivision of the available bandwidth results in poorer axial resolution, but in this instance, the net effect is a decrease in low-contrast lesion detectability.[38] Frequency compounding (otherwise known as integrated backscatter imaging) would appear to be equivalent to simple low-pass filtering in the axial direction, using a bandwidth equal to that used for one of the components in the compound image.[55]

Nonlinear Filtering

Many nonlinear filtering procedures have been explored in the past, meeting (at best) with limited success. Median filtering,[56] which is well known as an edge preserving noise smoothing process, performs poorly with speckle noise.[34,57] In a process known as homomorphic filtering, a logarithmic transform converts multiplicative noise to additive noise, permitting conventional methods such as smoothing or Wiener filtering to be applied before inverting the logarithmic transform.[26,34] A better performer (on SAR images) in this category seems to be a rather ad hoc approach known as the geometric filter, which smooths fine detail more than it does spatially correlated or large-amplitude structures and may be suitable for A-mode processing.[58]

Adaptive Processing

Adaptive filtering techniques have been regarded in SAR imaging as comparatively successful,[59–63] particularly when combined with some degree of diversity processing.[64] Such filters only smooth the image where local image statistical evidence indicates the occurrence of speckle artifact. Substantial interest has arisen in applying similar approaches to medical echographic images,[65–73] and the early indications in this field are also promising. Medical ultrasound systems, however, impose a considerable amount of processing on the echo signal, and if the unprocessed signal is not available, it is important to ensure that the statistical measures used to recognize speckle are independent of machine characteristics as well as the mean scattering level.[74] When implemented in this manner, local adaptive smoothing (LAS) appears to provide promising results in terms of the trade-off between improvement in speckle SNR and loss of spatial resolution, although an improvement in target detectability has yet to be demonstrated.

As mentioned earlier, image filtering may be regarded as a special case of spatial diversity. It is interesting here to speculate that if adaptive control is successful for this compounding method, it also may be used advantageously with other approaches to compounding. As an example of what is achievable, Figure 5-3 illustrates, using the same image sets as for Figure 5-2, the results for single-frame LAS and for adaptively controlled temporal compounding. The use of true three-dimensional data sets is likely to improve further the performance of LAS.

Signal Reconstitution

There are two quite different approaches to signal reconstitution, both of which in some sense attempt to recover information that would appear to have been lost during the image-forming process.

Deconvolution may be regarded as an approach to speckle reduction because it attempts to "unfold" some of the overlapping target reflections that have interfered to produce the speckle pattern.[65] It relies on the image being a simple convolution of the pulse and beam with the backscattering impulse response of the tissue[10] and must be implemented before demodulation or other signal processing. Therefore, it would not work effectively if much of the speckle resulted from other mechanisms such as multiple scattering or phase cancellation in the receiver. In practice, the phase aberrations that result from propagation in inhomogeneous media and the speed of computation limit applicability of this method at present.[32] In microwave imaging, side lobe artifacts and associated speckle have been reduced by a processing method known as CLEAN, which successfully subtracts the point spread function of the receiver centered first on the brightest targets and progresses iteratively through less bright targets to the noise level.[75]

Envelope reconstruction is an intriguing approach that attempts to make use of instantaneous phase discontinuities (or large frequency excursions) in the A-line, obtained from its Hilbert transform, to recognize local occurrences of destructive interference.[76,77]

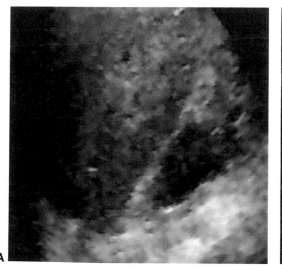 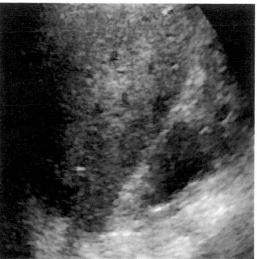

Fig. 5-3 (A) Image of Figure 5-2A processed by local adaptive smoothing. **(B)** Image set used to produce Figure 5-2B, processed using a new technique of adaptive frame averaging.

Several alternative schemes for applying corrective measures at such signal locations are under development by this group of authors. One of these offers the attractive prospect of reconstructing the envelope that would have existed if the destructive interference had not taken place by combining an additive local correction (at the point of cancellation) with the original envelope. The method is said to be suitable for real-time implementation. Its limitations have not been fully explored yet, but it would seem reasonable to expect some kind of compromise to be necessary between effective detection of all true points of destructive interference and the occurrence of false-positive frequency excursions. The images processed using this approach may look different to compounded and filtered images, in which it is assumed that the tissue scattering information is in the mean or median echo level, because emphasis is being placed on the information in the peaks of the echo envelope (which represent constructive interference).

APPLICATIONS

Clinical Trials

Any discussion of the applications of speckle reduction at present must be somewhat speculative because no current widely available ultrasound systems incorporate speckle reduction processing other than temporal compounding, and neither the applications nor benefits of this have been evaluated. Angle compounding became a thing of the past when displaced by real-time imaging, but examples of experience in this earlier phase of clinical ultrasound (e.g., lists of diagnostic criteria best observed in compound or simple scans of the breast[78] suggest that (because of the compromises already discussed) it will remain desirable, for sometime at least, to be able to switch between the various types of image display. Temporal processing is in effect used in this way at present, and some of

the preliminary studies reviewed confirm this viewpoint.

The greatest published clinical experience specifically of speckle reduction methods is with LAS, although all trials to date have been of a preliminary nature, involving relatively small numbers of cases. By collating the opinions of observers, it was concluded[79] that images processed with an adaptive median filter were visually acceptable and often preferred to the original images for overall quality and depiction of structures of interest. A fast on-line processing system has been used[80] with an algorithm that incorporated corrections for the effects of signal processing in the ultrasound scanners[74] to conduct several clinical trials. A quantitative evaluation was conducted of the effects of speckle reduction on echograms of breast masses and space-occupying liver disease by asking experienced radiologists to score visually 14 of the image features known to be most useful for distinguishing malignant from benign solid breast masses[81] and other features more generally important in ultrasound assessment of malignancy (e.g., the clarity of anatomic information, textural detail, lesion margins, relative echo level, and attenuation).[82] These reports (83 liver and 71 breast examinations) indicated that LAS resulted in no apparent loss of significant anatomic detail and a net reduction of image artifacts. Although the visual descriptions of some of the diagnostic criteria for breast masses were altered, in most cases it became easier to assess such features. Image information in general was remarked as being seen better in nearly 50 percent of cases and worse in only 8 percent of cases. In another trial, the image structures removed or preserved by LAS of 20-MHz B-scans of skin tumors were compared with the histologic structures present on stained sections of the tumors after excision. This confirmed that LAS is a useful aid to image interpretation, leading to an apparently correct understanding of which image details truly correspond to resolved tissue structure.[83] From a study of 64 patients, it was concluded[84] that LAS helps by enhancing B-scan textural changes and may be particularly useful for improving accuracy in the visual classification of diffuse liver disease, a result that now has been confirmed by an independent study (A.E.A. Joseph and D.K. Nassiri, personal communication). Finally, it has been concluded[85] that the reduction in gray-level variance and improvement in perceived boundary definition brought about by LAS make it a desirable step before analyzing regional myocardial backscattering amplitude and estimating areas such as of the left ventricular cavity.

Discussion of Applications

In general, most of the studies just described suggest that speckle reduction makes ultrasound images easier to interpret. Possible consequences of this, now requiring evaluation, are improved observer performance (diagnostic accuracy), decreased observer variability, shorter reading times, easier training of observers, and reduced variation in observer performance from one machine to another.

LAS may be used as a route to tissue characterization using B-mode texture parameters.[83,84] Appropriate choice of the function that relates the measured echo texture properties to the smoothing bandwidth of the filter results in what might be termed a *textural emphasis filter*, which could be a visually more acceptable alternative to the direct viewing of texture parametric images as investigated by others.[86] Such an approach has parallels in radar image processing, where the use of segment-dependent image smoothing is sometimes preferable to displaying the segmented image directly.[87]

Speckle reduction, in one form or other, is also likely to be a prerequisite for more effective application of many previously used postprocessing operations[57] (e.g., amplitude windowing, histogram manipulation, false-color encoding, and edge enhancement). It is not likely that attempts to improve contrast resolution using color,[87] for example, will have much impact until the limiting factor of speckle noise is first dealt with. Pseudocolor also may be used to improve quantitative comparability between image regions,[88,89] but at present, such methods tend to enhance the perception of speckle noise by converting the fluctuating echo intensity into rapid color changes. Application of edge enhancement without speckle reduction tend to emphasize the speckle at least as much as other high spatial frequency components of the image. The ability of speckle reduction to improve boundary definition[82,85] suggests that it should have a role in improving automatic contouring[90] and surface detection for area/volume and reduction of artifacts in displays generated by three-dimensional rendering techniques.[91]

CONCLUSIONS

Contrast discrimination is an important determinant of echographic image quality, influencing disease detection and diagnosis, but it is currently limited by the existence of coherent speckle noise. Among the improvements in instrument performance that can be anticipated in the coming years, it is likely that some of the most significant progress will result from the incorporation of hardware and software to take advantage of one or more of the many speckle reduction methods now available. It will then be possible, through clinical experience, to evaluate the usefulness of reduced speckle imaging in terms of the likely benefits discussed in this chapter.

ACKNOWLEDGMENTS

The author is grateful to the U.K. Cancer Research Campaign and Medical Research Council for research program funding.

REFERENCES

1. Hill CR, Bamber JC, Crawford DC et al: What might image echography learn from image science? Ultrasound Med Biol 17:559, 1991
2. Climent V, Carpinell JP: Reduction of temporal contrast sensitivity due to presence of speckle. J Optic (Paris) 19:15, 1988
3. Lowe J, Bamber JC, Webb S, Cook-Martin G: Perceptual studies of contrast, texture and detail in ultrasound B-scans. SPIE Med Imaging II 914:40, 1988
4. Wagner RF, Insana MF, Brown DG et al: Texture discrimination: radiologist, machine and man. p. 310. In Blakemore C (ed): Vision, Coding and Efficiency. Cambridge University Press, Cambridge, 1990
5. Trahey GE, Hubbard SM, Fischer TA, von Ramm OT: Angle independent blood-flow mapping using B-mode images. Ultrason Imaging 10:70, 1988
6. Bamber JC, Hasan PK, Cook-Martin G, Bush N: Imaging of tissue dynamics and low velocity blood flow using B-scan decorrelation rate. Br J Radiol 61:537, 1988
7. Arsenault HH: International Conference on Speckle. SPIE 556, 1985
8. Burckhardt CB: Speckle in ultrasound B-mode scans. IEEE Trans Sonics Ultrason 25:1, 1978
9. Abbott JG, Thurstone FL: Acoustic speckle: theory and experimental analysis. Ultrason Imaging 1:303, 1979
10. Bamber JC, Dickinson RJ: Ultrasonic B-scanning: A computer simulation. Phys Med Biol 25:463, 1980
11. Flax SW, Glover GH, Pelc NJ: Textural variations in B-mode ultrasonography: a stochastic model. Ultrason Imaging 3:235, 1981
12. Dainty JC: Laser Speckle and Related Phenomena. 2nd Ed. Springer, Heidelberg, 1984
13. Wagner RF, Smith SW, Sandrik JM, Lopez H: Statistics of speckle in ultrasound B-scans. IEEE Trans Sonics Ultrason 30:156, 1983
14. Oosterveld BJ, Thijssen JM, Verhoef WA: Texture of B-mode echograms: 3-D simulations and experiments of the effects of diffraction and scatterer density. Ultrason Imaging 7:142, 1985
15. Wilhelmij P, Denbigh P: A statistical approach to determining the number density of random scatterers from backscattered pulses. J Acoust Soc Am 76:1810, 1984
16. Tuthill TA, Sperry RH, Parker KJ: Deviation from Rayleigh statistics in ultrasonic speckle. Ultrason Imaging 9:81, 1988
17. Rath U, Schlapps D, Limberg B et al: Diagnostic accuracy of computerized B-scan texture analysis and conventional ultrasonography in diffuse parenchymal and malignant liver disease. J Clin Ultrasound 13:82, 1985
18. Nicholas D, Nassiri DK, Garbutt P, Hill CR: Tissue characterization from ultrasound B-scan data. Ultrasound Med Biol 12:135, 1986
19. Bamber JC, Nassiri DK: Spatial resolution and information content in echographic texture analysis. IEEE Ultrason Symp Proc 937, 1986
20. Insana MF, Wagner RF, Garra BS et al: Supervised pattern recognition techniques in quantitative diagnostic ultrasound. SPIE Pattern Recognition Acoustical Imaging 768:146, 1987
21. Wagner RF, Insana MF, Brown DG, Smith SW: Statistical physics of medical ultrasound images. SPIE Pattern Recognition Acoustical Imaging 768:22, 1987
22. Guenther BD, Nichols G, Christensen CR, Bennett JS: Speckle noise and object contrast. p. 202. In Shaw R (ed): Image Analysis and Evaluation. Society of Photographic Scientists and Engineers, Washington, DC, 1977
23. Lee JS, Grunes MR, Mango SA: Speckle reduction in multipolarization, multifrequency SAR imagery. IEEE Trans Geosci Rem Sens 29:535, 1991
24. Shankar PM, Newhouse VL: Speckle reduction with improved resolution in ultrasound images. IEEE Trans Sonics Ultrason 32:537, 1985
25. Smith SW, Wagner RF, Sandrik JM, Lopez H: Low contrast detectability and contrast/detail analysis in medical ultrasound. IEEE Trans Sonics Ultrason 30:164, 1983
26. Lim JS, Nawab H: Techniques for speckle noise removal. Opt Eng 20:472, 1981
27. Foster FS, Patterson MS, Arditi M, Hunt JW: The conical scanner: a two transducer ultrasound scatter imaging technique. Ultrason Imaging 3:62, 1981
28. Robb RA: A software system for interactive and quantitative analysis of biomedical images. p. 333. In Hohne KH, Fuchs H, Pizer

SM (eds): 3-D Imaging in Medicine. NATO ASI Series Vol. F60. Springer, Berlin, 1990

29. Collet Billon A, Le Guerinel Y, Rua Ph: 3D echography. p. 55. In: Revue Annuelle LEP. Laboratoires d'Electronique Philips, Limel-Brevannes, 1989

30. Cunningham JJ, Bacani M: Reduced-speckle imaging. Appl Radiol (Jan/Feb):91, 1985

31. Sommer FG, Sue JY: Image processing to reduce ultrasonic speckle. J Ultrasound Med 2: 413, 1983

32. Harris RA, Follett DH, Halliwell M, Wells PNT: Ultimate limits of ultrasound imaging resolution. Ultrasound Med Biol 17:547, 1991

33. Wells PNT, Halliwell M: Speckle in ultrasonic imaging. Ultrasonics 19:225, 1981

34. Jain AK, Christensen CR: Digital processing of images in speckle noise. SPIE Applications Speckle Phenomena 243:46, 1980

35. Parker DL, Pryor AT: Analysis of B-scan speckle reduction by resolution limited filtering. Ultrason Imaging 4:108, 1982

36. Kossoff G, Garrett WF, Carpenter DA et al: Principles and classification of soft tissues by grey scale echography. Ultrasound Med Biol 2:89, 1976

37. Trahey GE, Smith SW, von Ramm OT: Speckle pattern correlation with lateral aperture translation: experimental results and implications for spatial compounding. IEEE Trans Ultrason Ferroelect Freq Contr 32:257, 1986

38. Trahey GE, Allison JW, Smith SW, von Ramm OT: Speckle reduction achievable by spatial compounding: experimental results and implications for target detectability. SPIE Pattern Recognition Acoustical Imaging 768: 185, 1987

39. Ohya A, Yuta S, Shimazaki T, Nakajima M: Speckle reduction by compact spatial compounding system. Jpn J Med Ultrason 18:1, 1991

40. Silverstein SD, O'Donnell M: Speckle reduction using correlated mixed-integration techniques. SPIE Pattern Recognition Acoustical Imaging 768:168, 1987

41. Holm HH: Ultrasonic scanning in the diagnosis of space occupying lesions of the upper abdomen. Br J Radiol 44:24, 1971

42. Carson PL. Scherzinger AL, Bland PH et al: Ultrasonic computed tomography instrumentation and human studies. p. 187. In Jellins J, Kobayashi T (eds): Ultrasonic Examination of the Breast. Wiley, Chichester, 1983

43. Hiller D, Ermert H: Ultrasound computerized tomography using transmission and reflection mode: application to medical diagnosis. p. 553. In Ash EA, Hill CR (eds): Acoustical Imaging. Vol. 12. Plenum Press, New York, 1982

44. Shattuck DP, Weinshenker MD, Smith SW, von Ramm OT: Explososcan—a parallel processing technique for high-speed ultrasound imaging with linear phased-arrays. Proc SPIE 535:247, 1985

45. Kerr AT, Patterson MS, Foster FS, Hunt JW: Speckle reduction in pulse echo imaging using phase insensitive and phase sensitive signal processing techniques. Ultrason Imaging 8:11, 1986

46. Smith SW, von Ramm OT: The Maltese cross processor: speckle reduction for circular transducers. Ultrason Imaging 10:153, 1988

47. Fink M, Mallart R, Laugier P, Abovelkaram S: A generalized framework for incoherent pulse echo processing and imaging: the random phase transducer approach. p. 121. In Lee H, Wade G (eds): Acoustical Imaging. Vol. 18. Plenum Press, New York, 1991

48. Entrekin R, Melton HE: Real-time speckle reduction in B-mode images. Proc IEEE Ultrason Symp 169, 1979

49. Magnin PA, von Ramm OT, Thurstone FL: Frequency compounding for speckle contrast reduction in phased array images. Ultrason Imaging 4:267, 1982

50. Gehlbach SM, Sommer FG: Frequency diversity speckle processing. Ultrason Imaging 9:92, 1987

51. Yoshida C, Nakajima M, Yuta S: Real time speckle reduction in ultrasound echo imaging. p. 544. In Gill RW, Dadd MJ (eds): Proc 4th Meeting of the World Fed Ultrasound Med Biol. Pergamon Press, Sydney, 1985

52. Singh S, Tandon SN, Gupta HM: Ultrasonic speckle reduction using FM pulses. Proc 8th Ann Conf IEEE Eng Med Biol Soc 3:1059, 1986

53. Ohya A, Yuta S, Akeyama I et al: Speckle noise reduction using PM pulses. p. 295. In Shimizu H, Chubachi N, Kushibiki J (eds): Acoustical Imaging. Vol. 17. Plenum Press, New York, 1989

54. Galloway RL, McDermott BA, Thurstone FL: A frequency diversity process for speckle reduction in real-time ultrasonic images. IEEE Trans Ultrason Ferroelectr Freq Contr 35:45, 1988

55. Thomas LJ, Barzilai B, Perez JE et al: Quantitative real-time imaging of myocardium based on ultrasonic integrated backscatter. IEEE Trans Ultrason Ferroelect Freq Contr 36:466, 1989

56. Hall EL: Computer Image Processing and Recognition. Academic Press, New York, 1979

57. Yokoi H, Tatsumi T, Ito K: Quantitative colour ultrasonography by means of computer aided simultaneous tomogram. Ultrasonics 13:219, 1975

58. Crimmins T: Geometric filter for speckle reduction. Appl Opt 24:1438, 1985

59. Lee JS: Speckle analysis and smoothing of synthetic aperture radar images. Comput Graph Image Proc 17:24, 1981

60. Lee JS: A simple speckle smoothing algorithm for synthetic aperture radar images. IEEE Trans Syst Man Cybern 13:85, 1983

61. Frost VS, Stiles JA, Shanmugam KS et al: An adaptive filter for smoothing noisy radar images. Proc IEEE 69:133, 1981

62. Li C: Two adaptive filters for speckle reduction in SAR images by using the variance ratio. Int J Rem Sens 9:641, 1988

63. Dewaele P, Wambacq P, Oosterlinck A et al: Comparison of some speckle reduction techniques for SAR images. p. 2417. In: Remote Sensing Science for the Nineties, Vol. 3. IEEE, Piscataway, 1990

64. Lee JS, Grunes MR, Mango SA: Speckle reduction in multipolarization, multifrequency SAR imager. IEEE Trans Geosci Rem Sens 29:535, 1991

65. Dickinson RJ: Reduction of speckle in ultrasound images: theory and application. p. 213. In Ash E, Hill CR (eds): Acoustical Imaging. Vol. 12. Plenum Press, New York, 1982

66. Bamber JC, Daft C: Adaptive filtering for reduction of speckle in ultrasound pulse-echo images. Ultrasonics 24:41, 1986

67. Bamber JC, Cook-Martin G: Texture analysis and speckle reduction in medical echography. SPIE Pattern Recognition Acoustical Imaging 768:120, 1987

68. Castellini G, Labate D, Masotti L et al: An adaptive Kalman filter for speckle reduction in ultrasound images. J Nucl Med Allied Sci 32:208, 1988

69. Loupas T, McDicken WN, Allan PL: An adaptive weighted median filter for speckle suppression in medical ultrasonic images. IEEE Trans Circ Syst 36:129, 1989

70. Greiner T, Loizou Ch, Pandit M et al: Speckle reduction in ultrasonic imaging for medical applications. p. 2993. In: Int Conf Acoust Speech Signal Processing. IEEE, Piscataway, 1991

71. Koo JI, Park SB: Speckle reduction with edge preservation in medical ultrasonic images using a homogeneous region growing mean filter (HRGMF). Ultrason Imaging 13:211, 1991

72. Bamber JC, Phelps JV: A real-time implementation of coherent speckle suppression in B-scan images. Ultrasonics 29:218, 1991

73. Tsao J, Itoh T: Reduction of speckle in ultrasound B-scans by adaptive filtering. Proc Jpn Soc Ultrasound Med 279, 1988

74. Crawford DC, Bell DS, Bamber JC: Implementation of ultrasound speckle filters for clinical trial. p. 1589. In McAvoy BR (ed): 1990 Ultrasonics Symposium Proc. IEEE, Piscataway, 1991

75. Tsao J, Steinberg BD: Reduction of sidelobe and speckle artefacts in microwave imaging: the CLEAN technique. IEEE Trans Ant Prop 36:543, 1988

76. Leeman S, Seggie DA: Speckle reduction via phase. SPIE Pattern Recognition Acoustical Imaging 768:173, 1987

77. Forsberg F, Healey AJ, Leeman S, Jensen JA: Assessment of hybrid speckle reduction algorithms. Phys Med Biol 36:1539, 1991

78. Jellins J, Reeve TS, Kossoff G: Breast pathology as demonstrated by ultrasound. p. 25. In Leopold R (ed): Ultrasound in Breast and Endocrine Disease. Churchill Livingstone, New York, 1984

79. Loupas T, Allen PL, McDicken WN: Clinical evaluation of a digital signal-processing device for real-time speckle suppression in medical ultrasonics. Br J Radiol 62:761, 1989

80. Bamber JC, Bell DS, Crawford D et al: Fast image processing systems for evaluating the clinical potential of ultrasound speckle

suppression and parametric imaging. SPIE Med Imaging III: Image Processing 1092:33, 1989

81. Crawford DC, Tohno E, Stepniewska K et al: The effect of speckle reduction on breast echography. p. 131. In Kasumi F, Ueno E (eds): Topics in Breast Ultrasound. Shinohara, Tokyo, 1991

82. Crawford DC, Cosgrove DO, Tohno E et al: The visual impact of adaptive speckle reduction on ultrasound B-mode images. Radiology 183:555, 1992

83. Bamber JC, Crawford DC, Bell DS et al: Effects of speckle reduction processing on ultrasound B-mode images of skin tumours. p. 447. In Ermert H (ed): Acoustical Imaging. Vol. 19. Plenum Press, New York, 1992

84. Bleck JS, Gebel M, Hebel RH et al: Intelligent adaptive filter in the diagnosis of diffuse and focal liver disease. p. 375. In Ermert H (ed): Acoustical Imaging. Vol. 19. Plenum Press, New York, 1992

85. Massay RJ, Logan-Sinclair RB, Bamber JC, Gibson DG: Quantitative effects of speckle reduction on cross sectional echocardiographic images. Br Heart J 62:298, 1989

86. Verhoeven JTM, Thijssen JM: Improvement in lesion detection by echographic imaging processing. p. 427. In Ermert H (ed): Acoustical Imaging. Vol. 19. Plenum Press, New York, 1992

87. Nguyen PY, Stamon G: Radar image processing for remote sensing. p. 315. In Levialdi S (ed): Digital Image Analysis. Pitman, London, 1984

88. Pizer SM, Zimmerman JB: Colour display in ultrasonography. Ultrasound Med Biol 9: 331, 1983

89. Logan-Sinclair R, Wong CM, Gibson DG: Clinical application of amplitude processing of echocardiographic images. Br Heart J 45: 621, 1981

90. Rouvrai B: Method and device for generating images from ultrasonic signals obtained by echography. U.S. Patent 4729019, March 1, 1988

91. Hohne KH, Fuchs H (eds): 3D Imaging in Medicine; Algorithms, Systems, Applications. Springer, Berlin, 1990

6

Three-Dimensional Imaging

Leonardo Masotti
Riccardo Pini

Like other medical imaging modalities such as computed tomography (CT) and magnetic resonance imaging (MRI), ultrasound has the theoretic possibility to generate three-dimensional images. The visualization of internal organ image data in three dimensions can reveal new information to aid physicians in diagnosis, volume calculation, and surgical planning. So far, however, only limited clinical applications have been reported[1,2] because of some technical limitations of currently available echographic systems and physical characteristics of ultrasound.

Because ultrasound is attenuated strongly by air, it is impossible to move the transducer around the human body as in CT scanning as this would not provide a good probe–skin coupling. The use of water path could solve the problem of coupling between patient and probe, but in many cases it requires cumbersome systems.

In echocardiography, the limited acoustic windows restrict even more the acquisition of sufficient two-dimensional tomographic images for three-dimensional reconstruction of the heart. Therefore, three-dimensional echographs must be based on new acquisition techniques specifically designed to solve the ultrasound physical problems. Furthermore, for imaging moving organs such as the heart, the acquisition time with traditional imaging is so short that the process is accompanied by loss of information. In 1953, Howry et al.[1] and, in 1967, Brown[3] described pulse-echo three-dimensional ultrasound scanners, but these were too slow for practical clinical use. High-speed ultrasound volumetric data acquisition systems will be the ultimate solution.[4,5]

SCANNING METHODS

To obtain a three-dimensional reconstruction by ultrasound, multiple two-dimensional images with known spatial orientation must be acquired. The scanning technique can be similar to CT (i.e., multiple parallel two-dimensional tomographic planes) to study small parts such as the breast, which can be immersed in a water bath while the transducer is connected to a computerized unit.[6] When studying organs that only can be visualized through limited acoustic windows, the three-dimensional reconstruction must use nonparallel two-dimensional images with known spatial orientations. Transducers locating systems have included a mechanical arm with position sensors (Fig. 6-1)[7–10] or an acoustic ranging device with multiple fixed microphones and spark gaps attached to a freely movable ultrasound transducer (Fig. 6-2).[11–13] These methods have limited clinical applicability, however, because they do not acquire a sufficient number of two-dimensional images to reconstruct three-dimensional echograms with the same spatial resolution as the original two-dimensional images. Moreover, discontinuities appear in the data when the reconstructed images result from contributions of adjacent portions acquired at different distances from the transducer, depending on the particular scanning mode adopted. The axial and lateral resolutions depend on the depth in the tissue. The axial resolution varies with the depth because the tissues selectively absorb the ultrasound energy so that the received echo signal has a bandwidth decreasing with increasing distance. Furthermore,

the lateral resolution (i.e., beamwidth) varies with the distance from the transducer even if electronic focusing is adopted.

In echocardiography, normal identification and tracing of endocardial borders or other interfaces are needed in each two-dimensional image, a tedious process that has precluded routine use of this technique. Finally, three-dimensional representations provided by this methodology, independently of the transducer location system adopted, are wire-frame models of the heart cavities or valves rather than realistic images.

Recently, methods have been proposed to acquire two-dimensional tomographic images for the three-dimensional reconstruction of the heart using transesophageal probes.[14] These systems have the advantage of displaying two-dimensional images with high definition, but the probe can be moved up and down and tilted in the esophagus only in a limited range, thus (but only rarely) preventing the acquisition of a sufficient number of tomographic images for a realistic three-dimensional reconstruction.

Because of the enormous clinical interest in angioplasty, echo catheter probes have been developed (Fig. 6-3)[15,16] that also can be used for acquiring data for three-dimensional im-

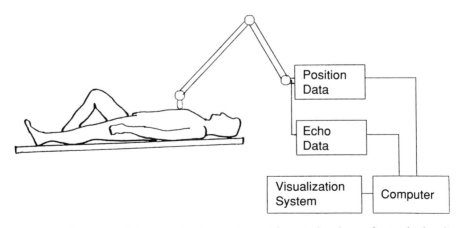

Fig. 6-1 Three-dimensional data acquisition system with articulated arm for probe localization.

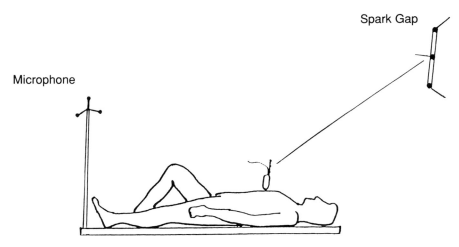

Fig. 6-2 Three-dimensional data acquisition system with acoustic technique for probe localization.

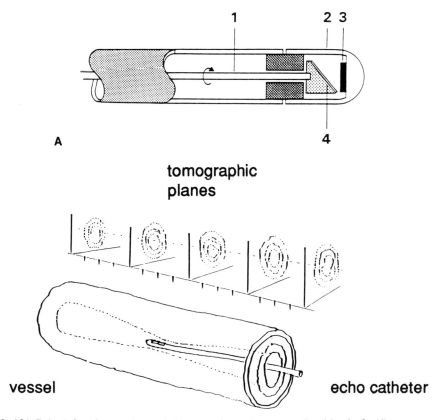

Fig. 6-3 **(A)** Principle of a mechanical driven echo catheter: (*1*) flexible shaft; (*2*) transparent dome; (*3*) transducer; (*4*) rotating mirror. **(B)** Three-dimensional display capability of an echo probe. (Fig. A from Bom and Roelandt,[15] with permission. Fig. B from Aretz et al.,[16] with permission.)

ages. In this case, the probe acquires two-dimensional sector or circular images in several parallel planes; by combining the images and the probe position information, three-dimensional images can be obtained by using sophisticated computer reconstructions. Recently, off-line three-dimensional reconstructions have also been extended to obstetrics[10] and ophthalmic applications.[17]

To perform three-dimensional reconstructions with the same spatial resolution as the original two-dimensional tomographic images, several possibilities have been proposed. For example, two-dimensional sector scans can be obtained with mechanical or phased array probes, combined with a third direction of sequential scanning (Fig. 6-4).[18–21] These systems have the advantage of acquiring a large number of tomographic images (typically more than 50), and they do not need a cumbersome external reference system.

Compared with other locating systems, the rotating transducers have the advantage of using an internal reference system, thus allowing an immediate check of the probe stability during the entire acquisition, whereas the mechanical arm and the acoustic range techniques do not record any changes in the patient position. In fact, with the rotating transducers, if the probe maintains the same relative position to the heart during the entire examination, the 0- and 180-degree images are mirror images. With this acquisition process, the volume close to the central axis is oversampled compared with the area near the image boundaries, so that the three-dimensional matrix does not have a uniform spatial resolution.

To avoid the movement of mechanical parts to select different two-dimensional tomographic planes, two-dimensional arrays have been proposed (Fig. 6-5).[4] Theoretically, with a two-dimensional phased array, it

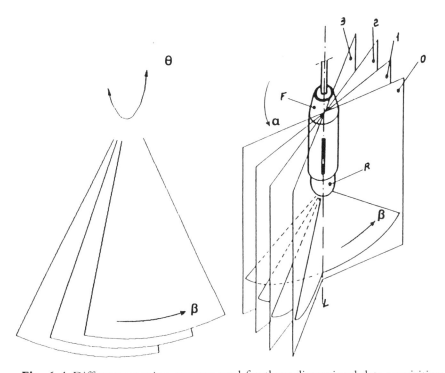

Fig. 6-4 Different scanning systems used for three-dimensional data acquisition.

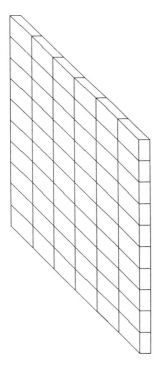

Fig. 6-5 Two-dimensional phased array.

that the problem of having a maximum frame rate (i.e., images per second) limited by the acquisition time is exacerbated when the number of scan lines is increased for volumetric imaging systems in real-time.

REAL-TIME THREE-DIMENSIONAL DATA ACQUISITION

A high-speed volumetric ultrasound imaging system[5] could solve the problem of the limitation in frame rate caused by the low propagation speed of ultrasound and the large number of scan lines of three-dimensional imaging. An unconventional solution for the transmitting and receiving mode processing has been introduced in the two-dimensional phased array system, the Explososcan,[4] incorporating parallel receive mode processing; multiple image scan lines are obtained for each transmit pulse. The basic idea is to design a transmit beam angular response sufficiently wide to include many narrower receive beams angularly centered about the transmit direction, thus making it possible to simultaneously receive many scan lines for each transmit pulse. In the two-dimensional phased array, a set of piezoelectric elements in a cross is used in transmission, and a different set of piezoelectric elements, again in a cross, is used in the receiving system. The received signal could be sent in parallel, after preamplification, to N different channels, one for each of the receiving directions. Thus N volumetric scan lines would be obtained for each transmit pulse, and the data acquisition rate would be increased by a factor of N.

would be possible to visualize different scanning planes by steering the ultrasound beam in any particular direction in the three-dimensional space. The extension of the one-dimensional phased array technology to two-dimensional arrays presents many practical limitations. To maintain good spatial resolution, a matrix of at least 64×64 elements must be realized[22] if the total transducer aperture is to be equivalent to the currently available two-dimensional sector-scan probes. This goal represents a challenging task with the present technology; one of the most advanced two-dimensional phased arrays presently being developed has 16×16 elements.[5]

The design and realization of the electronic integrated circuits and the electrical connections to the many (4,096 for the 64×64 square matrix) piezoelectric elements are very difficult tasks. Moreover, ultrasound has a relatively low propagation speed, so

In the Explososcan technique, the parallel receive processing system is simplified with respect to this solution. The simplified parallel receive processing is realized by the addition of small tapped delay line at the outputs of the main delay system for each receive channel. In this implementation, multiple delay processing channels are not required. The tapped delay lines introduce a linear progression of delay increments required to shift the receive beam by small increments away from the transmit direction. By changing the transmit set of piezoelectric elements or the setting of the transmit delay from a transmit pulse to the subsequent one, or both, the transmit direction is controlled; the receive set of piezoelectric elements and the setting of the delay processing channels are changed appropriately to obtain the different scan lines centered about the transmit direction. In principle, assuming that N is equal to the number of the scan lines of a two-dimensional tomographic image, with this technique the acquisition time for a two-dimensional tomographic image would be comparable with that required for each scan line in a conventional two-dimensional imaging system. Thus a volumetric scan consisting of a number of two-dimensional tomographic images comparable with the number of scan lines in a conventional two-dimensional imaging system would require a time compatible with real-time data acquisition of a beating heart (about 30 to 40 ms).

The system is complex, and the transmit beamwidth compatible with many parallel processed scan lines would imply a poorer lateral resolution than that obtained using focusing also for the transmit beam. A three-dimensional real-time ultrasound acquisition system with good geometric resolution, comparable with that of the present conventional two-dimensional images, is a long way from practical realization.

THREE-DIMENSIONAL IMAGE RECONSTRUCTION

Independent of the transducer locating system adopted for three-dimensional data acquisition, the reconstruction of three-dimensional images from multiple two-dimensional tomographic planes requires the implementation of a digital scan converter to obtain a cube of information in Cartesian coordinates. Systems based on hand-controlled scanning (e.g., mechanical arm or acoustic ranging devices) usually have the disadvantage of irregular scanning, with the large part of the final three-dimensional matrix being undersampled (Fig. 6-6). Thus, these systems do not permit the reconstruction of realistic three-dimensional images but only wire-frame models of the anatomic structures.

The scans obtained with a rotating transducer have a regular format that permits the reconstruction of a three-dimensional matrix with the same spatial resolution as the original two-dimensional images. This scanning procedure, however, leads to an oversampling around the axis of rotation; the scan conversion algorithm must be designed to avoid image artifacts. To obtain three-dimensional images with acceptable spatial resolution, the two-dimensional images must be digitized typically with 512×512 pixels and 256 gray levels. Thus, the three-dimensional matrix reconstructed by the scan converter would have a resolution of $512 \times 512 \times 512$ voxels or 128 megabytes.

To reconstruct three-dimensional images of the beating heart, at the present state of the art, at least an entire cardiac cycle must be acquired for each two-dimensional scanning plane with electrocardiograph synchronization. From the multiple two-dimensional images visualizing the heart at each specified time in the cardiac cycle, a three-dimensional matrix is reconstructed that represents the three-dimensional image at that time (Fig. 6-7). Because the frame rate ranges from 25 to 30 frames per second, 25 to 30 three-dimensional matrices must be reconstructed, with a total amount of digital information of more than 3 gigabytes. To process and store this amount of data requires a computer with large memory and very high speed.

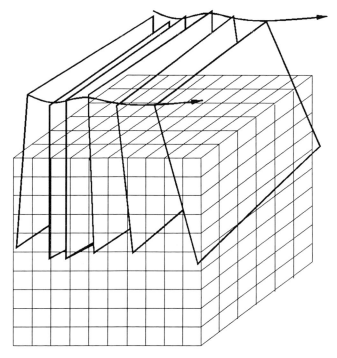

Fig. 6-6 Tomographic planes and parallelepiped data set.

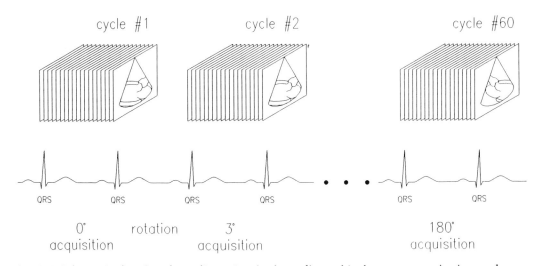

Fig. 6-7 Schematic showing three-dimensional echocardiographic data sequences in time and space.

IMAGE VISUALIZATION

To display three-dimensional data sets, multiple two-dimensional tomographic images with any spatial orientation can be selected or perspective projections can be created.[5] As already explained, if the three-dimensional matrix has been reconstructed from a sufficient number of two-dimensional images, the two-dimensional tomographic planes derived from the three-dimensional images have the same spatial resolution as the original two-dimensional echograms.[2] Moreover, the two-dimensional images can be derived with any spatial orientation allowing the visualization of tomographic planes that otherwise only can be obtained with CT or MRI. Finally, the simultaneous visualization of several slices can improve the understanding of complex anatomic structures.[22]

To create perspective projections, surface modeling techniques have been used.[9,18–20] Because the boundaries between soft tissues are often fuzzy, however, automatic segmentation procedures are difficult to implement and manual identification is a time-consuming process. Thus, volume rendering techniques that do not require data segmentation seem to be more easily applicable to three-dimensional echography. The algorithm used to create three-dimensional images is based on a technique called *ray tracing*,[23] modified to visualize three-dimensional fields. The light source and viewer's location are specified, and a simulation of the light propagation in the environment is then executed.[24] From the observer's viewpoint, in any given direction (or ray) a light intensity that depends from the light source position and the material properties of the voxels intercepted by the ray is received. Thus, in this visualization process, a crucial step is the assignment of material properties (i.e., reflectivity and transparency) to each voxel in the three-dimensional matrix.

Preliminary results suggest the possibility of combining volumetric rendering and surface modeling techniques to reveal fine details in three-dimensional echography using color-coded voxels.[22]

FUTURE PROSPECTS

Within a few years, it should be possible to package a computer with a scanner to achieve three-dimensional image acquisition and visualization without the penalty of decreased portability. Furthermore, it should be possible to reconstruct three-dimensional images of blood velocity jets so that their actual spatial orientations can be defined correctly.

REFERENCES

1. Howry DH, Posakony GJ, Cushman CR, Holmes JH: Three-dimensional and stereoscopic observation of body structures by ultrasound. J Appl Physiol 9:304, 1956
2. Pini R, Monnini E, Masotti L et al: Echocardiographic three-dimensional visualization of the heart. p. 263. In Hohne KH, Fuchs H, Pizer SM (eds): 3D Imaging in Medicine. Springer, Berlin, 1990
3. Brown TG: Visualization of soft tissues in two and three dimensions—limitations and development. Ultrasonics 5:118, 1967
4. Galloway L, Thurstone FL: Recent applications of parallel processing techniques to improve ultrasound B-mode images. Ultrason Imaging 8:69, 1986
5. von Ramm OT, Smith SW, Pavy HG: High-speed ultrasound volumetric imaging system. Parts I and II. IEEE Trans Ultrason Ferroelect Freq Contr 38:100, 1991
6. Itoh M, Yokoi H: A computer-aided three-dimensional display system for ultrasonic diagnosis of a breast tumor. Ultrasonics 17:261, 1979
7. Geiser EA, Christie LG, Conetta DA et al: A mechanical arm for spatial registration of

two-dimensional echocardiographic sections. Cathet Cardiovasc Diagn 8:89, 1982

8. Sawada H, Fujii J, Kato K et al: Three-dimensional reconstruction of the left ventricle from multiple cross sectional echocardiograms value for measuring left ventricular volume. Br Heart J 50:438, 1983

9. Raichlen JS, Trivedi SS, Herman GT et al: Dynamic three-dimensional reconstruction of the left ventricle from two-dimensional echocardiograms. J Am Coll Cardiol 8:364, 1986

10. Levaillant JM, Rotten D, Collet Billon A et al: Three-dimensional ultrasound imaging of the female breast and human fetus in utero: preliminary results. Ultrason Imaging 11: 149, 1989

11. Moritz WE, Pearlman AS, McCabe DH et al: An ultrasonic technique for imaging the ventricle in three dimensions and calculating its volume. IEEE Trans Biomed Eng 30:482, 1983

12. Linker DT, Moritz WE, Pearlman AS: A new three-dimensional echocardiographic method of right ventricular volume measurement: in-vitro validation. J Am Coll Cardiol 8:101, 1986

13. King DL, King DL, Yi-Ci Shao M: Evaluation of in vitro measurement accuracy of a three-dimensional ultrasound scanner. J Ultrasound Med 10:77, 1991

14. Martin RW, Bashein G, Detmer PR, Moritz WE: Ventricular volume measurement from a multiplanar transesophageal ultrasonic imaging system: an in-vitro study. IEEE Trans Biomed Eng 37:442, 1990

15. Bom N, Roelandt J: Early and recent intraluminal ultrasound devices. p. 85. In Gus-senhoven WJ, Bom N, Roelandt J (eds): Intravascular Ultrasound. Kluwer, Dordrecht, 1989

16. Aretz HE, Martinelli MA, LeDet EG: Intraluminal ultrasonic guidance of transverse laser coronary atherectomy. p. 153. In Gus-senhoven WJ, Bom N, Roelandt J (eds): Intravascular Ultrasound. Kluwer, Dordrecht, 1989

17. Yaremko MM, Dumke AE, Silverman R et al: Three-dimensional ultrasonic tissue characterization and imaging. Ultrason Imaging 11:150, 1989

18. McCann HA, Sharp JC, Kinter TM, McEwan CN: Multidimensional ultrasonic imaging for cardiology. Proc IEEE 76:1063, 1988

19. Ghosh A, Nanda NC, Maurer G: Three-dimensional reconstruction of echocardiographic images using the rotation method. Ultrasound Med Biol 8:655, 1982

20. Raqueno R, Ghosh A, Nanda NC et al: Four-dimensional reconstruction of two-dimensional echocardiographic images. Echocardiography 6:323, 1989

21. Pini R, Monnini E, Masotti L et al: Echocardiographic computed tomography of the heart: preliminary results. J Am Coll Cardiol 13:224A, 1989

22. Hottier F, Collet Billon A: 3D echography: status and perspective. p. 21. In Hohne KH, Fuchs H, Pizer SM (eds): 3D Imaging in Medicine. Springer, Berlin, 1990

23. Whitted T: An improved illumination model for shaded display Comm ACM 23:343, 1980

24. Greenberg DP: Light reflection models for computer graphics. Science 244:166, 1989

7

Needle Guidance Techniques

W. Norman McDicken

Of all the medical imaging techniques, ultrasound imaging is probably the most suited to the guidance of biopsy needles. The real-time display allows the needle tip to be observed as it is passes through tissues.[1,2] The small dimensions of ultrasound transducers and needles enable them to be used in conjunction both externally and internally on the patient. The small diameters of needles (e.g., 0.71 mm for a 22-gauge needle or 1.22 mm for 18-gauge) mean that the tissue sampling procedure can be repeated several times with little discomfort and negligible hazard to the patient. By directly assisting in the acquisition of specific tissue samples that are analyzed with all the resources of a pathology laboratory, ultrasound needle guidance often contributes to a quick, accurate, and detailed diagnosis. This technique may remove the need for tissue characterization by ultrasound or other types of imaging in many situations. However, because it is not strictly noninvasive, it cannot be used for serial examinations.

The value and acceptability of needle biopsy methods have resulted in their being widely applied to sample tissue from all soft tissue organs in the abdomen. This includes extensive use for amniocentesis, chorion villus sampling, and follicle aspiration in obstetrics and gynecology. The technique also has applications that are less easy to describe collectively, such as sampling the thyroid and parathyroid glands or the brain through a burr hole in the skull.

Ultrasound is used in the guidance of fine needles (20-gauge and 22-gauge) to collect cells for cytologic examination and with histology needles (18-gauge and 16-gauge), which extract small cores of tissue. The small cores of tissue provide sufficient material for further analyses to be used in addition to the cytologic assessments possible on fine needle samples. Examples of these analyses are histologic and immunologic tests, as well as electron microscopy. The biopty gun is a new tool of major significance for the acquisition tissue samples using histology needles[3] (Fig. 7-1). The gun is proving popular because it provides better tissue samples both in quantity and in quality. Good specimens are obtained by operators with a wide

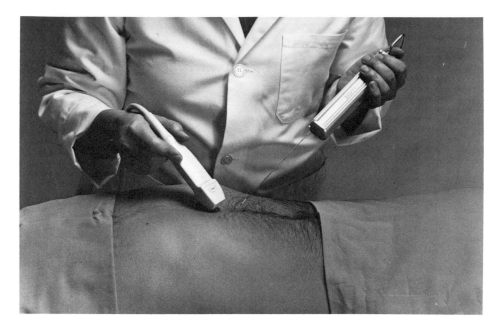

Fig. 7-1 Freehand-held arrangement of biopty gun and ultrasound transducer.

range of experience, as a consequence of the automated action. The noncutting ends of the needle and its stylet are clamped on compressed spring attachments within the body of the gun. The needle and stylet then are advanced into the tissue to within a specified distance from the site of interest (e.g., 1 or 2 cm). Release of the spring attachments rapidly injects the stylet, which has a recess in its side near the tip, farther into the tissue, followed virtually simultaneously by the outside needle. This double action cuts a core from the tissue that remains stationary because of its inertia. In an ultrasound department carrying out abdominal biopsy procedures, the biopty gun approach typically may be used two or three times as often as the fine needle one.

Although this discussion concentrates on tissue sampling, which is the most common procedure, ultrasound guidance is well suited to other techniques, such as the guidance of catheters, the injection of liquid or contrast material, the sampling of blood from a specific vessel or even the fetus, and the implantation of drainage devices.

ULTRASOUND SCANNER/NEEDLE COMBINATIONS

If during imaging the needle makes an angle to the ultrasound beam direction of less than about 60 degrees, the echo scattered from the irregular structure of the tip is observed in the ultrasound image. When the beam-to-needle angle is closer to 90 degrees, the echo from the smooth body of the needle becomes larger than that from the tip. Taking care to distinguish tip from body echoes, a needle in the tissue may be identified in an ultrasound image, permitting guidance of it to a desired location.

There are four conventional approaches to guiding a needle with an ultrasound scanner (Fig. 7-2). In Figure 7-2A, the scanner is used merely to locate the region of interest. In Fig-

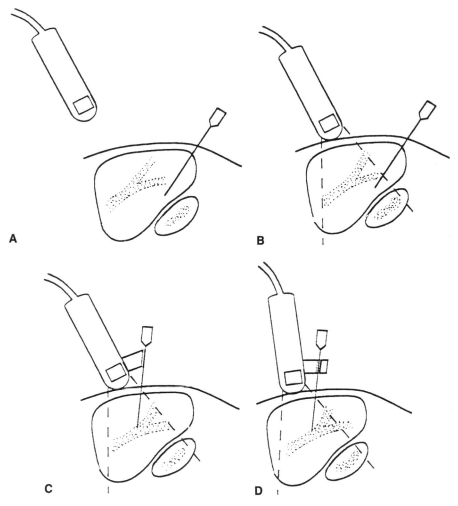

Fig. 7-2 Four conventional approaches to guiding a needle with an ultrasound scanner. **(A)** Prior visualization; **(B)** freehand tracking; **(C)** alignment with transducer; **(D)** guidance channel.

ure 7-2B, the scanner is used to track the needle tip as it is passed through the tissues. Because there is no fixed linkage between the transducer and the needle, the operator is required to exercise manual dexterity and spatial awareness. Although this freehand method is the most difficult, it is also popular because its flexibility allows adjustments necessitated by patient movement. The freehand approach also is commonly used with biopty guns. To define the needle path relative to the scanner, a simple approach involves moving the needle next to the side of

the transducer (Fig. 7-2C). A common precise technique uses a guidance channel attached to or within the transducer and through which the needle is passed into the body (Fig. 7-2D). In recent years, guidance channels have become widely available for application with internal transducers, in particular for follicle aspiration and chorion villus sampling (Fig. 7-3). Means for gathering biopsy samples also have been introduced with flexible ultrasound/optical endoscopes.

Many guidance channel attachments have

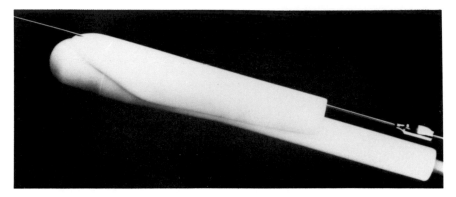

Fig. 7-3 Transvaginal transducer with a needle in its guidance channel. (Courtesy of Philips Medical Systems, London, England.)

been marketed over the years, and many have been ill suited to the task. The simplicity of the technology belies its value and often may have resulted in a less than rigorous approach to its development. Successful implementation of guidance techniques requires suitable instrumentation and skill on the part of the user. In the learning stage, benefit can be obtained using a simple test phantom constructed from reticulated foam in a small water tank. Alternatively a commercial test phantom can be purchased for training (Diagnostic Sonar, United Kingdom; Dansk Fantom Service, Denmark).

NEEDLE TIP OBSERVATION

The statement that a needle tip can be observed in the scan plane needs some qualification. It is usually true if the image quality is good and the tissues do not generate strong echoes. However, if the tissues produce strong echoes or partially distort the scanning beam and so degrade the image, the needle tip can be difficult to see. Bending of thin needles out of the scan plane also may make their detection difficult. Somewhat surprisingly, the tips of fairly thick needles (e.g., 18-gauge [1.22-mm diameter] histology needles) also are difficult to image. The problem of identification does not seem to have been reduced by improvements in

image quality. It appears that improved beam focusing results in the needle tip moving more readily out of the slice thickness of scanned tissue. Obviously, it is desirable that invasive procedures should be carried out in a simple and positive manner without the uncertainty that arises when the needle tip is not precisely located.

Many fabrications have been explored in attempts to make needle tips more visible. Needles are produced commercially in which the tips are roughened by etching or scoring to make them scatter ultrasound in all directions. Scattering also is increased by replacing the stylet with one that has a screw thread on it or by putting holes in the side of the needle.[4,5] Most of these needles increase the detectability, but they do not represent a complete solution to the problem. Another approach to increasing scattering at the needle tip is to oscillate the stylet within the needle and so create microbubbles in an atraumatic manner.[6] Recently, it has been shown that the color-flow Doppler mode can be used to detect a needle that is made to oscillate by hand.[7] This method may be developed successfully, but it will depend on the needle being distinguished from the surrounding moving tissue. A further increase in technical complexity seems to be required to render needle tips visible. Two types of needles have been developed that generate signals when an ultrasound pulse strikes the tip. Normally, it is the central stylet wire that is made sensitive by attaching an ultrasound detector to it. During most procedures (e.g., blood or tissue sampling), the stylet is withdrawn after insertion and the needle tip then is more difficult to see.

One type of sonically sensitive needle has a small piezoelectric polyvinylidene difluoride (PVDF) element mounted near to the end of the needle stylet (Fig. 7-4A).[8–10] At present, a 20-gauge needle is commercially available for operation with one make of ultrasound scanner (Biosponder, ATL, Seattle, Washington) (Fig. 7-5). When a pulse is detected by the PVDF element, the direction of the scanning beam is noted, as is the time from transmission to reception of the ultrasound pulse. This time allows the distance along the beam from the transducer to the needle tip to be calculated. Commonly, a flashing marker then is superimposed on the image to indicate the position of the tip. An audible bleep signaling that the tip has been detected also can be of value because it removes the need for the operator to watch the screen continually during the procedure. In theory, the piezoelectric element could be made to emit an ultrasound pulse in response to detecting the transducer pulse as in a normal

transponder system, but this is unnecessary, as the detected signal can be passed electronically to the display.

A second type of needle has a crystal mounted on the noncutting end of the stylet (Fig. 7-4B).[11–13] When the ultrasound pulse strikes the tip of the needle and stylet, some of the sonic energy travels along the stylet to the crystal and generates a signal. Acoustic insulation ensures that only sound absorbed at the tip passes to the detector. The signal is larger than might be expected because the stylet acts as a wave guide. The propagation of the energy along the stylet wire is by various longitudinal and transverse wave modes that travel at different velocities. Therefore, the signal received at the piezoelectric crystal is complex. However, the theory of sound propagation in a wave guide is well understood, and there is good agreement between theoretic mode velocities and experimental measurement (Fig. 7-6).[14] In practice, a high-energy longitudinal pulse wave arrives first at the crystal, and this can be used reliably to localize the needle tip (Fig. 7-7). This type of sonically sensitive stylet can be manufactured reasonably easily, and because it is detachable from the crystal, it is inexpensive. Needles have been made in sizes ranging upward from 22-gauge.

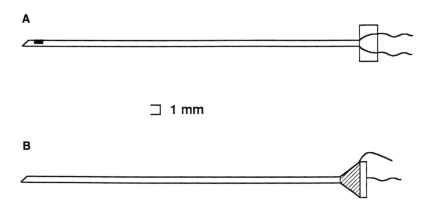

Fig. 7-4 Basic structure of two types of sonically sensitive biopsy needles. Examples use 22-gauge needles. **(A)** Piezoelectric element is near tip of stylet. **(B)** Piezoelectric element is in hand-held part of needle.

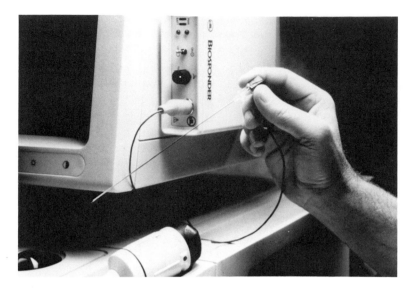

Fig. 7-5 ATL Biosponder with accompanying electronic box attached to scanner. (Courtesy of J. D. Aindow and J. Lesny.)

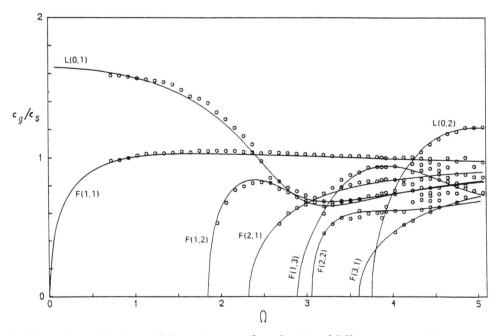

Fig. 7-6 Experimental points and theoretic curves for velocities of different wave modes in wire wave guides. Vertical axis is normalized group velocity and horizontal axis is frequency.

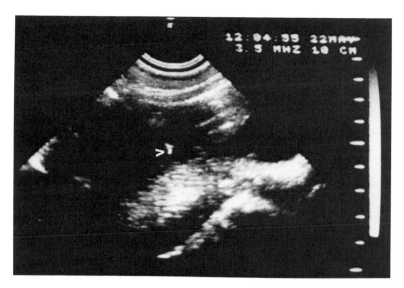

Fig. 7-7 Sonically sensitive needle in use for amniocentesis. Arrow indicates flashing marker spot superimposed on image at needle tip location.

The technology developed for sonically sensitive needles has not been incorporated yet into biopty guns.

STERILIZATION AND SAFETY

Sterilization is achieved by ethylene oxide treatment, although the time delay or lack of availability may make this difficult. Autoclaving is not recommended because it can damage the plastic or bonding of needles, guidance channels, or transducers. Disposable needles and guidance channels are commercially available; however, the latter only fit the transducers for which they have been designed. A sterile environment can usually be established by the use of sterile rubber sheaths or polythene bags to cover the transducer and part of or all the guidance channel. Sterile coupling liquid or electrocardiogram (ECG) jelly is also required. All these accessories have become commercially available.

Needle biopsy techniques, although invasive compared with other ultrasound ones, are relatively safe procedures. Several reviews have measured the risk. In a review of 11,700 fine needle biopsy procedures, the incidence of mortality was 0.008 percent, the major complication rate was 0.05 percent, and the total complication rate was 0.55 percent.[15] Seeding of the needle track with malignant cells is estimated to occur in approximately one patient in 21,000.[16] When amniocentesis was assessed in 7,238 Danish women for hazard, it was concluded that the risk of spontaneous abortion was approximately doubled in pregnancies in which the placenta was perforated and in those with blood-stained amniotic fluid.[17] The authors concluded that where there was a low risk of fetal abnormality, amniocentesis should be reconsidered if a placental perforation is unavoidable.

Although the biopty gun uses larger needles than those of fine needle biopsy, it is considered to be equally safe or possibly safer. This somewhat surprising result is due to the quick standardized action of the gun and the reduced number of passes required.[18]

FUTURE DEVELOPMENTS

The precision with which a needle can be guided ultrasonically to a specific site within the body means that this technique likely is to be used more in the future for investigation or treatment of disease at that site. Chemotherapy or radioactive agents may be injected to treat tumors. Likewise, laser or cryogenic therapy also is possible under ultrasound guidance.[19] Alcohol injection already is being investigated as a means of ablating parathyroid glands[20] and destroying metastases in the liver.[21]

REFERENCES

1. Otto RC, Wellauer J: Ultrasound-Guided Biopsy and Drainage. Springer-Verlag, Berlin, 1985
2. Holm HH, Kristensen JK: Ultrasonically Guided Puncture Technique. Munksgaard, Copenhagen, 1980
3. Lindgren PG: Percutaneous needle biopsy: a new technique. Acta Radiol 23:653, 1982
4. Rading CC, Charboneau JW, Felmlee JP, Meredith E: US-guided percutaneous biopsy: use of a screw biopsy stylet to aid needle detection. Radiology 163:280, 1987
5. Hurwitz SR, Nagoette MP: Amniocentesis needle with improved sonographic visibility. Radiology 171:576, 1989
6. Bisceglia M, Matala TAS, Silver B: The pump maneuver: an atraumatic adjunct to enhance US needle tip localization. Radiology 176:867, 1990
7. Kurohiji T, Sigel B, Justin J, Machi J: Motion marker in color Doppler ultrasound needle and catheter visualization. J Ultrasound Med 9:243, 1990
8. Lesny J, Aindow JD: Sonically-sensitive biopsy needles: the Dorchester approach. Br J Radiol 59:741, 1986
9. Aindow JD, Deogan DS, Robins P, Lesny J: Fine needle biopsy—enhanced visualisation using tip mounted miniature polymer transducers. Danish Society of Diagnostic Ultrasound: Proc 4th International Congress on Interventional Ultrasound, Copenhagen, 1986
10. Winsberg F, Mitty HA, Shapiro RS, Yeh H-C: Use of an acoustic transponder for US visualization of biopsy needles. Radiology 180:877, 1991
11. McDicken WN, Anderson T, Allan PA: The development of sonically-sensitive needles for biopsy by ultrasonic guidance. In Gill RW, Dadd MJ (eds): Proc 4th Meeting World Federation Ultrasound Medicine and Biology, Sydney, 1985
12. McDicken WN, Anderson T: Ultrasonic stylets for needles and catheters. Ultrasound Med Biol 10:L499, 1984
13. McDicken WN, Anderson T, MacKenzie WE et al: Ultrasonic identification of needle tips in amniocentesis. Lancet ii:198, 1984
14. Nicholson NC, McDicken WN, Anderson T: Waveguides in medical ultrasonics: an experimental study of mode propagation. Ultrasonics 27:101, 1988
15. Livraghi T, Damascelli B, Lombardi C, Spagnoli I: Risk in fine-needle abdominal biopsy. J Clin Ultrasound 11:77, 1983
16. Smith EH: The hazards of fine-needle aspiration biopsy. Ultrasound Med Biol 10:629, 1984
17. Kappel B, Neilsen J, Hansen KB et al: Spontaneous abortion following mid-trimester amniocentesis. Clinical significance of placental perforation and blood-stained amniotic fluid. Br J Obstet Gynaecol 94:50, 1987
18. Bernardino ME: Automated biopsy devices: significance and safety. Radiology 176:615, 1990
19. Charboneau JW, Reading CC, Welch TJ: CT and sonographically guided needle biopsy: current techniques and new innovations. AJR 154:1, 1990
20. Karstrup S, Holm HH, Torp-Pedersen S, Hegedus L: Ultrasonically guided percutaneous inactivation of parathyroid tumours. Br J Radiol 60:667, 1987
21. Livraghi T, Festi D, Monti F et al: US-guided percutaneous alcohol injection of small hepatic and abdominal tumors. Radiology 161:309, 1986

8

Techniques for Color-Flow Imaging

David H. Evans

Color-flow imaging (CFI) is the technique whereby a conventional ultrasound pulse-echo gray-scale image (representing cross-sectional anatomy) and a real-time color image (representing motion detected in the same scan plane) are combined to create a composite image that allows the investigator to visualize flow and anatomy simultaneously (Plate 8-1). The pulse-echo gray-scale component of the image, although not essential to producing a color-flow image, is invariably included, because it gives so much orientation information and its production is technically much less demanding than the Doppler color component. Although each pulse-echo image of tissue structure is, in principle, generated from the results of interrogating each sampling line through the tissue only once, to detect motion and generate the color image each sampling line must be sampled on several occasions and the change of phase of the received echoes, or the slight changes in the round-trip times between successive pulses, used to estimate the velocity of individual sample volumes away from or toward the transducer. In many ways, the Doppler part of CFI can be thought

of as the natural progression from multigate Dopplers, which allow the Doppler shift from many samples along a stationary ultrasound beam to be measured, but considerable advances in technology have been necessary to implement this step.

Before the development of CFI systems, several imaging systems based on Doppler detection had been built and described in the literature.[1-5] These devices used several continuous-wave (CW) and pulsed-wave (PW) techniques to generate either C-mode or B-mode images of blood vessels by systematically scanning through a single plane in the body and determining the presence or absence of flow in each tissue sample volume. They all, however, shared the same limitation, in that they required many seconds or, in some cases, several minutes of data to build up the complete image. The early devices simply recorded a bistable image where the presence of a Doppler signal above a threshold was written to the screen as a white pixel on a black background. Then the idea of color coding the display according to the velocity measured by the Doppler unit was introduced,[5] and it became possible to demonstrate stenoses in the carotid arteries as regions of increased flow velocity.

A particularly important step toward the modern CFI system was the combination of a multigate Doppler imaging system[6] with a pulse-echo B-scanner system.[7] The pulse-echo system was used to produce a monochrome image, which was then overwritten with color-encoded velocity information. To not blur the color image, each color line was acquired during the same part of several cardiac cycles; 20 to 30 cycles were required to complete the acquisition. The real breakthrough, however, occurred in 1982 when an autocorrelation technique for Doppler frequency estimation was introduced,[8,9] which permitted the estimation of mean velocity from a very short data segment and thus the real-time operation of a Doppler B-mode scanner.

CONFIGURATION OF CFI SYSTEMS

Figure 8-1 is a block diagram of the main components of a phase domain (PD) CFI system.[9,10] There are three processing paths, all of which take their input signal from the amplified received ultrasound signal. The conventional pulsed Doppler signal is obtained by gating the output of a pair of phase-quadrature demodulators and filtering the results. For display purposes, this signal is fast Fourier transformed, and the resulting spectra are displayed in the form of a sonogram. The information for the color display is also obtained from the output of the phase-quadrature demodulator but is digitized, filtered by delay line cancellers (DLC), and then used to calculate the velocity (and other derived quantities) at each point along the current color vector. The input for the gray-scale image is taken directly from the receiver out-

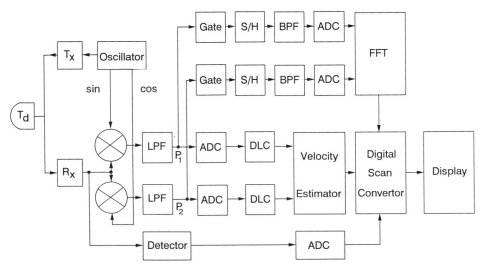

Fig. 8-1 Block schematic of a phase domain color-flow imaging system. Top processing path is for Doppler vector, middle path for color vector, and lower path for image vector. T_d, transducer; T_x, transmitter; R_x, receiver; LPF, low-pass filter; ADC, analog to digital convertor; DLC, delay line canceller; S/H, sample and hold; BPF, band-pass filter; FFT, fast Fourier transform.

put, and the signal amplitude at each point is suitably processed to form the image vector. Although the color and image vectors could be derived from the same pulses, it is usual to use separate pulses because the optimum length of an imaging pulse is shorter than that of a Doppler pulse.

All modern CFI systems use broadly similar processing pathways for the PW Doppler and image vector signals (although there is a trend to digitize the signals closer to the transducer), but as described later, some systems use a very different method for processing the color vector information,[11,12] which is usually called time domain (TD) processing or color velocity imaging.

TRANSDUCERS FOR CFI

There is some controversy among manufacturers as to which is the best type of transducer for CFI; but in principle, it is possible to use any of the varieties of transducer that are used for pulse-echo imaging (i.e., mechanical annular array transducers, phased arrays, or linear arrays), and each solution has its own advantages and disadvantages.

Mechanical Annular Arrays

The original CFI system made use of a mechanical annular array system, but most manufacturers have now abandoned this technology in favor of electronic beam steering methods. Perhaps the most important difference between the two technologies is that in the former the ultrasound beam is continuously swept through the tissue, whereas in the latter the beam moves through the tissue in several discrete steps.

Although the distinction between sweeping and stepping is of little consequence in pulse-echo imaging, where each image vector is interrogated only once, it raises several potential problems in CFI, because to measure velocity, it is necessary to interrogate each sample volume at least three times and often more (the reasons for this are explained later in the sections on signal processing). With a stepped system, each interrogating pulse for a particular color vector is transmitted in the same direction. With a swept system, this is not possible, and therefore even if there is no motion in the tissue, there is a reduction in the correlation between the successive sweeps used for each color vector that manifests itself as an increase in the noise of the frequency estimator. Another potential problem with a swept system is that the movement of the transducer during each acquisition period influences the measured Doppler shift frequency; the portion with the transducer moving toward the target measures a higher frequency shift than the portion with the transducer receding from the target. It has been argued, however, that the frequency spread this causes is equivalent to the frequency spread caused by sampling a finite length of a signal and that stepped systems suffer from exactly the same limitation.[13] Mechanical systems also require a finite amount of time to decelerate and accelerate at either extreme of their sweep, and this leads either to a change in line spacing or to a dead time, both wasteful of valuable acquisition time. This problem can be overcome by using a rotating transducer assembly, but this means that the sector angle cannot be traded off against frame rate.

Annular arrays also have several advantages over linear and phased array transducers. One particularly important feature is that they are able dynamically to focus both in the scan plane and transverse to the scan plane and thus to produce a narrow ultrasound beam. They also require fewer processing channels than the average phased array system, which means that the system is cheaper to manufacture and that the individual transducer elements have larger surface areas than those found in a phased array. This, in turn, means that more averaging of the ultrasound signals takes place at the transducer surface, which preserves more of the preamplifier dynamic range to deal with the large intrinsic dynamic range of the returning ultrasound signal. Finally, the swept nature of the ultrasound beam means that the high-pass delay line filters are easier to construct because the same initialization problems are not associated with a stepped transducer.

Phased Arrays

Like mechanical annular arrays, phased array systems produce sector scans, and therefore many of the merits and demerits of phased array systems compared with mechanical systems are implicit in the discussion in the previous section. Phased arrays, however, do have two advantages not yet discussed. The first is that they are physically smaller than mechanical sector scanners—this is clearly useful where only a small acoustic window is available. The second advantage, which applies to all electronically steered transducers, is that their ultrasound beams are agile (i.e., they are able to change direction almost instantaneously). This is a significant advantage when there is a requirement for simultaneous CFI and spectral Doppler or if the CFI is to use "interleaved sequence processing." In the case of simultaneous CFI and spectral Doppler, the ultrasound beam can be moved around in an optimal manner, first gathering part of a sector for CFI, then gathering some information from the sample volume chosen for the spectral Doppler display, then gathering some more data for the CFI, then back to the pulse-Doppler line, and so on. In interleaved sequence processing (as used by at least one manufacturer), several color vectors can be acquired simultaneously by firing the first pulse for the first vector, then the first pulse for the second vector and

so on for the third and fourth vectors, and then returning to fire the second pulse for each of the vectors and so on until the required number of pulses have been fired along each direction. The advantage of this technique is that when the bottom of the region of interest is relatively close to the transducer, the frame rate can be increased significantly.

Linear Arrays

The most obvious advantage of a linear array transducer when used for CFI is that it produces a series of parallel scan lines through the tissue, and therefore a straight vessel subtends the same angle to the ultrasound beam everywhere in the scan plane. This is not true for techniques that produce sector scans, where a straight vessel subtends different angles depending on its location. This effect is illustrated in Figure 8-2, where it may be seen that for a target moving with a constant velocity through the scan plane of a sector scan, the insonation angle changes continuously. At point A, the component of velocity the transducer measures is at a maximum toward the transducer; at point B, there is no component of velocity toward or away from the transducer and no motion is detected; at point C, the direction of the component of velocity relative to the transducer is opposite to that at point A. This effect is obviously most noticeable with vessels that lie roughly parallel to the skin surface, but it is a potential source of confusion for any vessel that crosses a significant number of scan lines.

The corollary of this effect for linear arrays is that if a vessel is parallel or nearly parallel to the skin surface (as is frequently the case for superficial vessels), it is possible for the Doppler angle to be 90 degrees at all points along the vessel if steps are not taken to steer the ultrasound beam away from a "vertical" direction. Therefore, most linear array systems designed for CFI have the ability to do

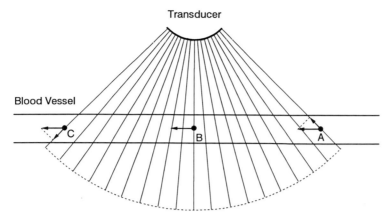

Fig. 8-2 Changes in components of velocity toward a transducer performing a sector scan, as a target moves with a constant velocity through the sector.

this using an electronic beam steering technique. Although this may go some way toward solving the problem, it is sometimes necessary also to include a triangular stand-off wedge between the transducer and skin surface to increase the angle further; this has obvious disadvantages of reduced sensitivity, awkwardness of use, and the possible creation of reverberation artifacts.

Perhaps the main disadvantage of linear array transducers, when compared with both mechanical annular arrays and phased arrays, is their relatively large "footprint." This means that they cannot be used flexibly in situations where a limited acoustic window is available.

SIGNAL PROCESSING

Before discussing CFI signal processing systems in any detail, it is instructive to compare the requirements for the Doppler processing in CFI systems with those for conventional PW and multigate Doppler systems. The fundamental difference between the two is that in CFI, to produce real-time images made up of a substantial number of image lines, only a limited number of ultra-sound pulses are available for the calculation of each velocity estimate. In the case of conventional Doppler systems, the sample time is limited only by the stationarity of the Doppler signal, which is of the order of 10 ms; this means that for a target at a depth of 50 mm (allowing a pulse repetition frequency [PRF] of up to 15 kHz), approximately 150 samples are available for each spectral estimation. By contrast, if the same target were studied with a CFI system using 64 lines with a frame rate of 15 frames per second, the maximum time available during each frame for interrogating the target would be 1 ms, giving at most 15 samples for analysis. This has important consequences both for the design of the high-pass filters required to reject stationary and near-stationary echoes and also for the design of the frequency estimation algorithms.

To understand the different approaches used to estimate velocity information from the ultrasound signal for CFI, it is necessary to appreciate the way in which conventional PW Doppler systems operate. This is different from the operation of CW systems, which directly compares the transmitted and received ultrasound frequencies to derive the

Doppler shift frequency. In the case of PW systems, although each pulse reflected from a moving target is Doppler shifted, with present technology it is difficult to measure the small shift (of the order of 0.01 to 0.1 percent of the transmitted zero-crossing frequency) because of the wideband nature of the short pulses necessary for good range resolution. Therefore, velocity is determined by comparing the phase of each successive reflected pulse with that of the master oscillator to reconstruct a "Doppler shift" waveform, which has exactly the same characteristics as a true CW Doppler shift waveform, from these successive phase shifts. In conventional PW systems, the rotation speed of the Doppler phase vector is estimated from about 100 pulses, usually with the aid of the fast Fourier transform (FFT), which provides the user with details of the distribution of target velocities. Unfortunately, such an approach is not viable for CFI systems because of the limited time available for interrogating each line through the tissue, and therefore, different methods have to be used to analyze the effects of motion on the received ultrasound pulses.

Two quite different approaches have been used to estimate target velocities for CFI, one based on measuring the phase differences between consecutively received echo signals (PD method) and one based on the time shifts between consecutive echoes (TD method).

PD Systems

The basic layout of a PD system is presented in Figure 8-1. Up until the output of the phase-quadrature demodulators (points P1 and P2), the signal path is substantially the same as for a standard PW Doppler system; from that point on, the paths diverge completely. The two channels for CFI are digitized and then passed to a pair of DLCs (also known as stationary echo cancellers or fixed target cancellers), which serve the same purpose in a CFI system as the "wall thump" filters in a conventional CW or PW Doppler

system (i.e., to reject the very high-amplitude echoes from stationary and near-stationary targets). Such a filtering technique is necessary, because although in principle it would be possible to achieve a similar end using many parallel processing channels (each filtering the signal from one sample volume), the large number of filters needed (perhaps 128 for each of the direct and quadrature signals) would be bulky and expensive.

Similarly, it would be possible, in principle, to use analog DLCs (e.g., as used in the infinite gate PW Doppler system[14]), but digital filters have the advantage of being much more flexible both in filter design and in accommodation of different PRFs as the maximum range of the color image is changed. A clear disadvantage of having to digitize the signals before the DLCs is that they have a much wider dynamic range than would otherwise be the case, and taken together with the requirement for high digitization rates, this is technically very demanding.

In essence, DLCs work by subtracting each successive echo signal from its predecessor. Signals arising from stationary objects are unchanged and thus cancelled, whereas signals from moving objects change and thus are preserved. This methodology is widely used in radar systems[15] and can be adapted to produce different frequency characteristics by allowing different degrees of feedback and cascading one or more stages. A general purpose single-stage DLC is shown in Figure 8-3A.

If the value of the feedback fraction, K, is set to zero, the filter has a finite impulse response; if K is set to a small negative value, the rejection of low frequencies is improved at the expense of an extended transient response. Even if no feedback is used to achieve a FIR filter, ringing can be a problem, particularly with step scan systems. The use of feedforward to increase the improvement

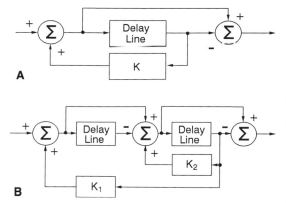

A

B

Fig. 8-3 Stationary echo cancellation circuits. **(A)** General purpose single-stage delay line canceller; **(B)** general purpose dual-stage delay line canceller. K, feedback fraction.

factor (defined as r_o/r_i, where r_o and r_i are the target-to-clutter ratios at the filter output and input, respectively, averaged over all target velocities[15]) can produce severe ringing, and steps may need to be taken to initialize the system for each new direction.[16]

Figure 8-3B shows a dual-stage DLC. Dual- and multiple-delay cancellers have wider clutter rejection notches than single-delay cancellers and, therefore, have an enhanced ability to reject not only echoes from stationary targets but also echoes from near-stationary targets. This can be important in CFI, particularly for targets such as the heart, where there may be very large echoes from moving solid structures that require rejection. The drawback of multiple-stage DLCs is that they reduce the signal-to-noise ratio (SNR) of the system because the effective number of independent pulses available for further processing is reduced. It is shown later that at least two independent pulses must be available before a velocity estimate can be calculated; this means that three pulses in total are needed for a single estimate using a single-stage DLC, four pulses are needed for a two-stage system, and so on. Although the increase in the number of pulses needed

for a single estimate may be insignificant if many pulses are available for analysis, CFI systems are sometimes required to produce estimates of velocity from only four or five pulses to achieve an acceptable scan area and frame rate, and such considerations may then become important. To calculate variance, at least four independent pulses are necessary, which is even more restrictive.

Unfortunately, whatever techniques are used, DLCs are unable to approach the sharpness of the filters used in conventional systems, and much of the art in building a good CFI system is in optimizing the stationary and near-stationary echo cancellation. Furthermore, it is known that the DLCs cannot be treated totally in isolation because they may introduce a correlated noise term into previously uncorrelated noise signals,[17] and because of this, the use of second-order infinite impulse response filters, which are said to reduce the bias from signals that have a poor SNR, has been recommended.

Once stationary echo cancellation has taken place, the filtered range phase signals are sent to the "velocity estimator." In CFI systems, the velocity estimator does not do a full spectral analysis of the Doppler signal from each pixel, but rather estimates parameters such as mean frequency and some measure of spectral spread. The reason for this is three-fold. First, when CFI was first introduced, real-time FFT of the information from each pixel was beyond the then state of the art for processing speed. Returning to the example given earlier in which a maximum time of 1 ms was available for sampling along each color vector, if this were split into only 64 pixels, there would still be only 16 μs available for each FFT. Modern digital signal processing chips can perform 16-point complex FFTs in approximately 50 μs, so that with some degree of parallel processing, a real-time FFT approach now, 10 years after the introduction of CFI, would be just about feasible using standard hardware.

A second reason for not performing spectral analysis is that the FFT, the classical method of obtaining signal spectra, has a frequency resolution limited to the reciprocal of the data segment analyzed and has an extremely large variance unless some averaging can be performed.[18] For the example quoted earlier, the best possible spectral resolution for the 1-ms data segment would be 1 kHz, and any windowing would degrade this. This limitation becomes less severe if the interleaved sequence processing (ISP) described earlier is used, because instead of acquiring one 1-ms data segment every 1 ms, fourfold ISP would allow the acquisition of four 4-ms data segments every 4 ms, the computational time restriction remaining unchanged. Modern spectral estimation techniques (e.g., autoregressive spectral analysis) have considerable advantages over FFT for the analysis of short data segments and have shown considerable promise as methods of analyzing Doppler signals[19–21] but require even more computational time than FFTs and cannot overcome the intrinsic noisiness of the Doppler data.

The third reason for not performing spectral analysis, one that will remain even when processing speeds increase further and better spectral analysis techniques can be applied in real-time, is simply the problem of displaying so much information. If spectra were calculated, they could be stored for further processing (but then, so could the raw data even now; in either case the data storage requirements would be large). However, bearing in mind that each pixel represents a small sample volume within the tissue, all the operator requires from the CFI system is an indication of mean or maximum velocity and some indication of spectral spread, which may give some information about disturbed flow. If the operator then requires more detailed information about the flow in any particular region of the tissue, a region of interest can be defined and spectral analysis on the signal from that sample volume can be carried out.

Several methods have been suggested as being suitable for frequency estimation in multigate and CFI systems,[22–25] and any one algorithm may appear under different names in different places. Four basic algorithms that recur throughout the literature are described here: the zero-crossing detector, the phase detector, the instantaneous frequency detector (IFD), and the autocorrelator.[24]

ZERO-CROSSING DETECTOR

Zero-crossing detectors are frequently used in simple CW and PW Doppler systems because of their low cost and ease of construction, even though they are known to have several significant limitations.[26] They have also been used in multigate systems,[27,28] apparently with considerable success. They function by detecting each occasion on which either the "direct" or "quadrature" signal passes through zero, and from this information they estimate the root mean square frequency of the signal. This process is illustrated in Figure 8-4. The signal vector is rotating in a counterclockwise direction and the quadrature signal changes its sign from negative to positive between $t = t_2$ and $t = t_3$, the direct signal changes from positive to negative between $t = t_4$ and $t = t_5$, and the quadrature signal goes negative again between $t = t_6$ and $t = t_7$. From these three zero-crossings, the only information available is that the phase of the signal vector has changed in a positive direction, by somewhere between 180 degrees and 360 degrees in six sample periods, and thus the frequency is between $\frac{1}{6}T$ and $\frac{1}{12}T$, where T is the sampling period. With a large number of zero-crossings, a reasonable estimate of frequency should be possible, but because of the timing considerations associated with CFI systems, more than 16 samples seldom are available for analysis, and usually far fewer, and under these circumstances, the zero-crossing detector is not a viable system. At low velocities and particularly when few data samples are

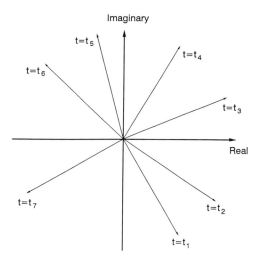

Fig. 8-4 Successive positions of a signal vector relative to real and imaginary axes as it rotates in a counterclockwise direction.

available, there may be no zero-crossings at all. From this discussion, it appears that what is needed for CFI systems are techniques that measure the angles between successive signal vectors, so that small phase changes can be detected, and this is precisely how the rest of the frequency estimation systems described here do operate.

PHASE DETECTOR

Estimators based on the "phase detector" algorithm or part of it[24] have appeared under different names including "phase detector,"[29,30] "infinite gate,"[14] "I/Q algorithm,"[31] and "double correlation centroid detector."[22] The basis of the technique can be simply explained with reference to Figure 8-5, which shows the positions of a signal vector during two successive samples, $(i - 1)$ and (i). The angular frequency, ω, of the vector is defined as its rate of change of phase, or

$$\omega = \frac{d\Phi}{dt}. \qquad (1)$$

The phase of the signal for sample i, Φ_i, is

simply the arctangent of $Q(i)/I(i)$ and substituting this into Equation 1 leads to the relationship

$$\omega = \frac{I(i)\dot{Q}(i) - Q(i)\dot{I}(i)}{I^2(i) + Q^2(i)} \qquad (2)$$

where a dot indicates a derivative with respect to time. If the derivatives are replaced by the finite backward differences between the samples (i) and $(i - 1)$[25] and the result is averaged over a number of samples, Equation 2 may be rewritten as

$$\bar{\omega} = \frac{1}{\tau} \frac{\displaystyle\sum_{i=1}^{N} I(i)Q(i - 1) - Q(i)I(i - 1)}{\displaystyle\sum_{i=1}^{N} I^2(i) + Q^2(i)} \qquad (3)$$

where τ is the pulse repetition interval. Figure 8-6 is a schematic representation of the signal processing path necessary to implement this algorithm.

The performance of the phase detector has been discussed by several authors.[24,25,31] Its most obvious drawbacks are that its frequency output only can be unambiguous over the range $\pm \pi/2$ radians (i.e., $\pm$PRF/4 or half the Nyquist frequency) and that, because of the squared terms in the denomi-

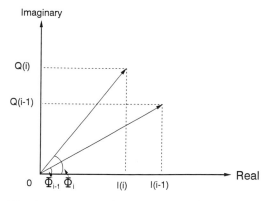

Fig. 8-5 Position of a rotating signal vector during two successive samples $(i - 1)$ and (i), showing in-phase components $I(i - 1)$ and $I(i)$ and quadrature components $Q(i - 1)$ and $Q(i)$.

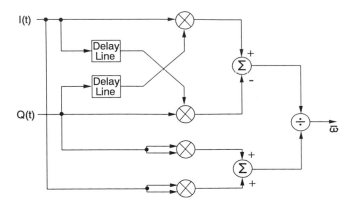

Fig. 8-6 Schematic representation of signal processing path necessary to implement the phase detection algorithm.

nator, the estimation is biased by any non-Doppler shifted components applied to the input. In theory, most nonshifted signals are removed by the DLCs, but inevitably some leak through, as does uncorrelated electronic noise. Both of these lead to an increase in the size of the denominator and a reduction in sensitivity to flow of the estimator. Simulation studies to evaluate the stationary and dynamic performance of the phase detection algorithm have also shown that its performance is rather poor.[24] Only with relatively narrowband signals (bandwidth ≤ 0.1 PRF) and SNRs of 30 dB or greater were acceptable values for the relative error obtained for center frequencies of up to 0.2 PRF. Either increasing the signal bandwidth or decreasing the SNR led to a rapid deterioration in the performance of the estimator.

INSTANTANEOUS FREQUENCY DETECTOR

The IFD apparently was first used in a multigate system.[6,32] Its basic operation can be explained by again making reference to Figure 8-5. The angular frequency can, as before, be written as the rate of change of phase (Equation 1), and this may be approximated by

$$\omega \approx \frac{\Phi_i - \Phi_{i-1}}{\tau}. \tag{4}$$

Both Φ_i and Φ_{i-1} may be written in terms of arctangents of the in-phase and quadrature signals, which, after averaging over several samples, N, leads to the following expression:

$$\overline{\omega} = \frac{1}{N\tau} \sum_{i=1}^{N} \left[\arctan \frac{Q(i)}{I(i)} - \arctan \frac{Q(i-1)}{I(i-1)} \right]. \tag{5}$$

Figure 8-7 is a schematic diagram of this algorithm. Simulations have been performed on this detector[24,28] that have shown its performance to be considerably superior to that of the phase detector. For narrow bandwidth signals with a high SNR, its output is unambiguous over a range of $\pm \pi$ radians (i.e., $\pm$PRF/2). As with the phase detector, the output of the IFD falls away when either the SNR decreases or the bandwidth increases. This is caused mainly by mapping of instantaneous frequencies outside the ± 0.5 PRF range back into the -0.5 to $+0.5$ interval. Because of this, its performance (and that of other PD detectors) also depends on the shape of the spectrum being processed. If the frequency spectrum is skewed so that the mean frequency is closer to the maximum frequency than would otherwise be the case (e.g., in spectra resulting from plug as opposed to parabolic flow), the performance of the IFD is better for a given mean frequency, because the maximum frequency is farther

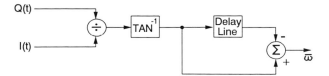

Fig. 8-7 Schematic representation of signal processing path necessary to implement the instantaneous frequency algorithm.

from the Nyquist frequency and fewer mapping errors occur.

The IFD also tends to overestimate velocity for very low Doppler frequencies (below approximately PRF/10 to PRF/20)[24] in exactly the same way as conventional CW and PW Doppler units[33]; the reason for this is that the high-pass filters (implemented by DLCs in CFI systems) remove not only the unwanted low-frequency clutter signals, but also the low-frequency blood flow signals.

THE AUTOCORRELATOR

The autocorrelator was the first frequency estimation technique applied to CFI[8,9] and is probably still the most widely used algorithm in CFI systems. Referring once again to Figure 8-5, it was shown in the previous section that the angular frequency could be written as the difference between the angles Φ_i and Φ_{i-1} and the pulse repetition interval (Equation 4). The tangent of an angle may be written as the ratio of the sine and cosine of the angle, that is,

$$\tan(\Phi_i - \Phi_{i-1}) = \frac{\sin(\Phi_i - \Phi_{i-1})}{\cos(\phi_i - \phi_{i-1})}. \quad (6)$$

The sines and cosines of angle differences can be expanded easily, so that Equation 6 may be rewritten as

$$\tan(\Phi_i - \Phi_{i-1})$$
$$= \frac{\sin \Phi_i \cos \Phi_{i-1} - \cos \Phi_i \sin \Phi_{i-1}}{\cos \Phi_i \cos \Phi_{i-1} - \sin \Phi_i \sin \Phi_{i-1}}. \quad (7)$$

If the sine and cosine terms are now expressed as the in-phase and quadrature magnitudes of the vectors and an average frequency calculated by summing over a number of pulses, Equation 7 may be rewritten as

$$\overline{\omega} = \frac{1}{\tau}\arctan\left\{\frac{\sum\limits_{i=1}^{n} I(i)Q(i-1) - Q(i)I(i-1)}{\sum\limits_{i=1}^{n} I(i)I(i-1) + Q(i)Q(i-1)}\right\}. \quad (8)$$

This algorithm is represented schematically in Figure 8-8. The numerator and denominator of the term in the brackets of Equation 8 are the imaginary and real parts of the complex autocorrelation of the Doppler signal evaluated for a single lag, and hence the name of this algorithm. Comparison of the derivation of Equations 5 and 8 leads to the conclusion that for a single pair of signal vectors, the outputs of the IFD and autocorrelator must be identical, and because of this, the estimators are often treated as being one and the same in the literature.[25,31] They differ, however, in the way the averaging of two or more results is performed, and the autocorrelator can be considered an improved design of the IFD.[24] Inspection of Equation 8 shows that noise that is uncorrelated from sample to sample and that is uncorrelated with the signal is smoothed out and does not contribute significantly to the denominator and that, therefore, the mean frequency estimate is unbiased.[25] This noise immunity has appeared in simulations[24] in which the autocorrelator provided an adequate estimate of the center frequency of the Doppler signal irrespective of whether the SNR was 30 dB or only 10 dB, although a decreasing SNR led to an increase in the variance of the estimate. Like

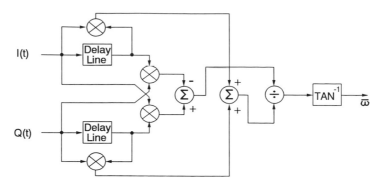

Fig. 8-8 Schematic representation of signal processing path necessary to implement the autocorrelation algorithm.

the IFD, the autocorrelator gave an unambiguous output for narrow bandwidth signals over the range of $\pm\pi$ radians (as would be expected from Equation 8). Furthermore, even for wide bandwidth signals (of up to 0.3 PRF), the autocorrelator output correctly tracked the mean frequency beyond 0.4 PRF. This is because the autocorrelator has the important property of correctly accounting for partial aliasing of a continuous spectrum.[24] Although the autocorrelator has a high immunity to uncorrelated noise, it is affected by correlated noise, and it has been pointed out[17,25] that DLCs inevitably introduce a correlated component into the noise. This means that the autocorrelator can be vulnerable to biasing by noise but that the level of bias can be reduced if IIR filters are used, and indeed with second-order infinite impulse response filters, the bias can be reduced close to zero.

Of the four PD estimators discussed, the autocorrelator has distinct advantages when compared with the other three frequency estimators. The zero-crossing detector requires a longer data segment than is normally available in CFI application. The phase detector can at best respond correctly to frequencies of $\pm$PRF/4, and even within this range it only functions well with high SNRs and relatively narrow bandwidth signals. The IFD performs considerably better than the zero-crossing detector and phase detector, and with a high SNR and a signal bandwidth of up to 0.1 PRF can give good results. The autocorrelator, however, outperforms the IFD on every front; it is less vulnerable to the effects of both noise and aliasing and, because of this, can satisfactorily cope with wideband signals.

TD Systems

The TD approach to CFI is quite different from that of the various PD methods so far described. It works directly on the RF A-lines rather than the demodulated signals, and it calculates the movement of the targets by detecting the time shift between successive range gated echoes by finding the maximum of their cross-correlation function, rather than calculating the phase shift between successive samples.[11,12,34,35] Figure 8-9, which should be compared with Figure 8-1, is a block diagram of the main components of a TD system. The PW Doppler vector path is identical to that in a PD system and therefore is indicated merely as an input to the digital scan converter. The color vector path, however, is completely different. The RF A-lines are digitized immediately after the receiving amplifier, and the processing is carried out digitally from then on. The signal is passed through a fixed echo canceller to remove echoes from stationary structures

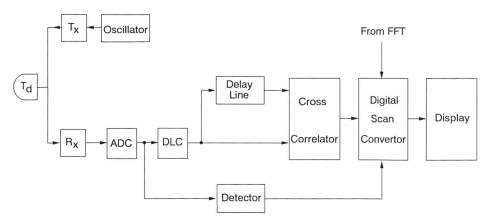

Fig. 8-9 Block schematic of a time-domain color-flow imaging system. Abbreviations are the same as those in Figure 8-1.

and then on to the cross-correlation unit, which consists of a further delay line and an algorithm for calculating the cross-correlation between the direct and delayed signals for a series of small negative and positive time shifts. Finally, the processor finds the maximum of the cross-correlation function and calculates velocity from the apparent displacement of the target that has occurred within the pulse repetition period.

The image vector path is nearly the same as in Figure 8-1, except that, as the RF signal has to be digitized for the CFI vector, the information needed for the image vector is also available in a digital form right at the beginning of the processing chain.

The TD method of obtaining color vector information is technically more demanding than the PD method because of the much higher digitization rate and data throughput necessary but is claimed to have significant advantages in accuracy, noise immunity, and lack of susceptibility to aliasing.

The argument concerning accuracy is that to obtain good spatial resolution it is necessary to use broadband (short-pulse) excitation of the transducer and that the shape of the resulting ultrasound pulses is significantly modified by frequency-dependent attenua-

tion and scattering in the tissues.[36–38] This pulse shaping has a significant effect on the mean frequency of the received pulses and thus biases the measured Doppler shift. The TD method, however, only measures time delays and therefore is not affected by the filtering effects of the tissues.[12] Despite this theoretic argument, which has frequently appeared in the literature, it is far from clear what effect frequency-dependent attenuation and scattering do have on the measurement of velocity when using PD techniques, and some authors[39,40] have gone so far as to suggest that they may be insignificant in practice.

The reason for the superior noise immunity of TD systems is claimed to be that PD systems are susceptible to the fluctuations of the local mean frequency of the ultrasound A-line, induced by the random interference between the echoes from the many scatterers within the tissues, whereas because TD systems are dependent only on times of flight and not frequency, they are not.[12] Practical TD systems do appear to produce estimates with much less variance, which means that fewer individual estimates need to be averaged to obtain each color vector. This in turn means that TD systems can work with a higher frame rate or a greater line density, or both, and that less interpolation is needed to produce acceptable image quality. Thus, in a comparison of the standard deviations of the estimates of the displacements of band-limited signals using both the complex autocorrelation algorithm and a correlation interpolation algorithm for different SNRs, the TD technique was found to be significantly less sensitive to the effects of noise.[41] It was also shown that the standard deviation did not vary significantly from the reciprocal of the square root of the number of samples used for either technique, as would be expected if the process corresponded to one of uncorrelated noise averaging.

The third advantage claimed for TD techniques is that because they measure time rather than phase they are not susceptible to aliasing. This may be the case when there is a strong signal and little noise, because the cross-correlation has an unambiguous global maximum. Because of the limited bandwidth of the signal and its consequent periodic nature, however, it seems likely that under low SNR conditions and when successive A-lines are derived from slightly different scatterer paths, there may be ambiguity about which correlation maximum to use and thus the appearance of aliasing. The aliasing properties of the correlation interpolation method have been shown to be very similar to those of the autocorrelator.[41]

An analysis[34] of the errors involved in the estimation of flow velocity profiles using TD correlation has shown that the precision of the method, P, defined as the standard deviation of the estimate of the time delay divided by the true time delay, τ_0, may be written

$$P = \frac{\sqrt{2}}{\beta \mu \tau_0 \text{SNR}} \quad (9)$$

where β is the RMS bandwidth of the received echoes and μ is the maximum correlation coefficient of the echoes without noise. Thus the precision of the estimate is inversely proportional to the product of the SNR and RMS bandwidth. It is also dependent on the time delay but not in an entirely simple way, because μ, the maximum correlation coefficient of the echoes, is also dependent on τ_0. This is because, as the time that elapses between successive interrogating pulses becomes greater (and thus the greater the value of τ_0 for a given velocity), the greater the number of scatterers that enter and leave the sample volume and, therefore, the smaller the value of the maximum correlation. Thus if the PRF is too low, the precision is poor because μ is small; if the PRF is too high, the precision is also poor because τ_0 is small. The same publication[34] also examined the errors associated with windowing, those associated with scatterers moving at different velocities within the range cell, those associated with the time duration of the system impulse response, and those associated with the intensity profile across the ultrasound beam. A companion paper[35] provided experimental verification of several effects related to measurement of volumetric flow using TD correlation.

At present, most CFI systems use PD techniques to derive their color vector information. It remains to be seen if the apparent advantages that TD systems offer with respect to noise immunity will be considered worth the added complication and expense of building such systems.

DISPLAY OF COLOR-FLOW IMAGES

The final common destination for all signals in the CFI system is the color display, although the PW Doppler signal may also be presented as an audible output. The color vector and image vector information are used to create the real-time color-flow image, whereas the conventional Doppler information derived from a selected sample volume is displayed in the form of a sonogram.

It is usually possible either to display the color image and the spectral Doppler sonogram separately or to display both simultaneously,[42] although the time sharing necessary to achieve this inevitably reduces the image frame rate.

The color-flow image consists of both anatomic and velocity information. Where the Doppler power is insignificant, the pulse-echo information is used to produce a conventional gray-scale image of the tissue; where the Doppler power is significant, the gray-scale image is suppressed and the Doppler information is written in a color-coded format.

Several schemes have been used to encode the color vector information, although most are based on the use of blue shades to represent blood moving away from the transducer and red shades to represent blood moving toward the transducer.[43] The earliest systems[10] encoded the magnitude of the mean velocity by the intensity of the two colors, with bright blue and bright red representing high velocities, typically away from and toward the transducer, respectively. The variance of the velocity estimate (indicating the bandwidth of the Doppler signal) was also displayed by adding green to the display, so that as bandwidth increased (caused by disturbed flow), the red shades tended to yellow and the blue shades tended to cyan. Another commonly used approach to color display is to encode the velocity information by color hue rather than intensity, although in this case, intensity may also vary at the same time. Whatever the system chosen, the display should include a color scale showing the range of colors being used, but the operator must not forget that CFI systems, like conventional Doppler systems, can measure only the component of velocity along the ultrasound beam.

An alternative to displaying velocity is to display the Doppler power in each pixel, and many machines now have a "power mode" display. For this type of display, blue and red are still used to indicate flow direction, but intensity is used to indicate Doppler power. Because the Doppler power represents the amount of flowing blood rather than its velocity, this has the advantage of being much less angle-dependent and can make image interpretation easier.

Most modern machines have several display options from which the operator can choose, together with an array of features that can alert the operator to possible aliasing, and permit the performance of many postprocessing operations, such as tagging selected velocities and acquiring time-averaged color images.

CURRENT AND FUTURE DEVELOPMENTS

CFI is still at a fairly early stage in its development, and considerable improvements and innovations can be anticipated over the next few years. Among these will almost certainly be new frequency estimation algorithms, methods for overcoming aliasing limitations, techniques that address the Doppler vector problem, and improved display techniques.

Frequency Estimation Algorithms

In some ways it is surprising what little progress has been made in this area during the past 10 years or, to put it another way, how good the autocorrelation method has proved to be when compared with other methods. The possibility of using low-order autoregressive modeling to estimate both mean frequency[44,45] and maximum frequency[44] has been discussed, and its use in the latter application may be of some considerable interest because current algorithms do not yield any measure of maximum frequency. Another approach that may have something to offer is that which exploits the effects of scatterer velocity on the signal delay and on the frequency shift.[46,47]

Antialiasing Techniques

Aliasing is the well-known phenomenon that occurs when the restrictions implicit in the sampling theorem[48] are not complied with (i.e., a signal is not sampled at a rate that is at least twice as high as its highest frequency component). If such undersampling does occur, there is inadequate information to reconstruct the signal properly, and the frequency components that are beyond the "Nyquist limit" (half the sampling frequency)[49] are interpreted incorrectly as lying within the Nyquist range. This is particularly easy to understand in pulsed Doppler and PD CFI systems, where the Doppler shift signal is reconstructed by examining the phase change that occurs between each successive transmitted pulse. Because phase is cyclic, if the Doppler shift frequency is not sampled sufficiently often, the phase change exceeds $\pm \pi$ radians but without additional information still must be interpreted as lying within this range.

The obvious solution to overcome aliasing is to sample the signal more frequently, but in pulsed Doppler applications, there is an upper limit to this because of the finite propagation time of ultrasound and because range ambiguity arises if an ultrasound pulse is transmitted before the previous pulse has had time to return from targets at the maximum range of interest. Although such depth ambiguity may be acceptable under some circumstances in conventional pulsed Doppler systems, it is clearly not so in CFI systems. Combining the requirements that the sampling frequency must be at least twice the maximum Doppler shift frequency and that each pulse must have time to return from the target before another is transmitted leads to a simple expression[50] for the maximum velocity, V_{max}, which may be detected un-

ambiguously at a range R:

$$V_{max} = \frac{c^2}{8RF_0} \tag{10}$$

where c is the velocity of ultrasound in tissue and F_0 is the carrier frequency. Substitution of some realistic values into this equation shows that aliasing can easily be a problem in CFI (e.g., if R is 7.5 cm and F_0 is 5 MHz, V_{max} is only 0.75 m/s), and this is particularly so when high-velocity flow needs to be imaged in deep structures (e.g., when imaging flow through a stenosed heart valve). Therefore, there is considerable interest in techniques for overcoming aliasing, and several approaches to this have been adopted.

The first attempts to overcome aliasing in Doppler ultrasound relied on the transmission of random and pseudorandom noise rather than tone bursts. A system that used continuous transmission of a random signal worked with simple targets but had difficulty coping with the complex target situation found in the body, where there are very large echoes from stationary structures.[50] The technique was improved by using bursts of pseudorandom noise, and it was claimed to be able to reduce range ambiguity by a factor of 2.[51] Unfortunately, commercial devices based on the use of random noise do not appear to have been built, which suggests that these techniques are of limited value in practice.

Consideration of the resolution of frequency aliases by making use of physiologic information (the continuity of flow and some knowledge of the direction or timing of the blood flow being interrogated, or both) introduced the idea of frequency tracking beyond the Nyquist limit.[52] Although it is usual to interpret all Doppler frequencies as lying between $-PRF/2$ and $+PRF/2$, if the bandwidth of the signal is strictly limited to less than PRF they can be interpreted as lying anywhere between f_x and $f_x + PRF$, where

f_x is a frequency determined using physiologic information. Thus, if it is known that flow in a certain vessel never reverses, f_x can be set at zero and frequencies anywhere between 0 and PRF can be dealt with satisfactorily. In CFI terms, this is the equivalent of "rotating the color map," so that instead of interpreting phase changes of between 0 radians and $-\pi$ radians as reverse flow, they are interpreted as rapid forward flow. Frequency tracking takes this concept one step forward, so that instead of fixing f_x, it is allowed to vary and is reset after each estimate of frequency f_e, as $f_e - PRF/2$. In this way, it is possible to track the signal successfully from estimate to estimate, provided that the changes between estimates are not greater than $\pm PRF/2$. Clearly, this system can only work if the true velocity is known at some point so it can be initialized appropriately, the most obvious point being diastole when the flow should be relatively low and the Doppler shift should be in the range between $-PRF/2$ and $+PRF/2$.

Frequency tracking has been applied more recently to multigate Doppler systems with some success[24,28] and is potentially useful in CFI systems, although there is more opportunity for a frequency change to exceed the critical range between two estimation sequences. In further development, the frequency is tracked along the spatial axis rather than the temporal axis, based on the assumption of continuity of the velocity profile along the beam direction.[53] This technique appears to work well on the bench and has advantages over the temporal axis technique in that it requires less storage, it is easy to initialize (because flow near to a vessel wall always should be relatively slow), each frame is independent (which means that it does not "miss" information while the ultrasound beam is interrogating other vectors), and errors are not automatically propagated into subsequent calculations.

One further antialiasing technique that has been suggested[54] relies on the use of two color-flow units working at different frequencies. Because the point at which each alias occurs depends on the carrier frequency (Equation 10), the interpretation of velocities that give rise to frequencies outside the $\pm PRF/2$ range is different depending on which transmitted frequency is used (Fig. 8-10). By combining the information from both carrier frequencies, it is possible to determine the value of the true velocity. The new Nyquist limit for such a combined system is determined by the difference between the carrier frequencies of the two channels, so that if 4- and 5-MHz carriers are used, the system has the aliasing characteristics of a system operating at 1 MHz. Early testing of a commercial system based on the dual frequency technique suggests that it might well be useful.[55]

It is fairly clear that several of the antialiasing techniques just described can operate well under simple test-bench conditions. It remains to be seen if they can be adapted to cope with the real aliasing problems in CFI (e.g., in the complex patterns that might arise from flow through a stenosed heart valve).

Vector Doppler Techniques

As with conventional Doppler systems, CFI systems can provide information only about the component of blood velocity along the axis of the transducer. This means that the measured velocity in any vessel, and hence its color coding, depends on the angle it makes with the transducer. This can be misleading, particularly if the blood vessel is roughly perpendicular to the ultrasound beam (see Fig. 8-2). Additionally, even if the operator takes great care in interpreting the Doppler information presented, assumptions must be made that may not necessarily be valid (e.g., that the flow in a vessel is parallel to its walls). Thus it would be most valuable

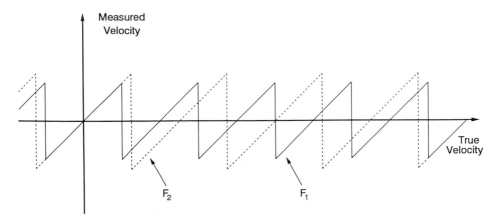

Fig. 8-10 Aliasing characteristics of two pulsed Doppler systems using slightly different carrier frequencies. F_1 is higher than F_2 and therefore produces higher Doppler shift frequencies for a given velocity. If both systems use the same pulse repetition frequency, the system with the higher carrier frequency aliases more frequently than that with the lower frequency. By combining information about the velocities measured with each of the systems, it is possible to calculate the true velocity even after a number of aliases have occurred.

if CFI systems were essentially angle-independent and able to measure both the magnitude and direction of flow in each pixel.

At least two separate approaches have been used to try to achieve angle-independent detection of motion. The first is based on the use of two or more Doppler transducers that interrogate each pixel from different angles and thus enable the true magnitude and direction of the velocity vector to be calculated. The second is based on the use of two-dimensional correlation searches applied to consecutively acquired images.

The first approach has been used by many investigators. For example, a set of three pulsed Doppler transducers located at three of the four corners of an equilateral tetrahedron has been used to determine the magnitude and direction of blood velocity vectors in the descending aortas of dogs.[56] Next, using a series of probes attached to the aortic arch of a dog, remarkable sets of velocity profiles from different sites during various phases of the cardiac cycle have been produced.[57] More recently, a (single sample volume) vector Doppler system has been tested on a human carotid artery with some success.[58]

The second approach is closely related to the TD approach to measuring velocity in CFI systems and is based on tracking the speckle pattern present on all ultrasound images.[59,60] A correlation search algorithm is applied to sequentially acquired images and the displacement vector between each "cell region," and the best correlated region in the subsequent image is taken to be the magnitude and direction of the target displacement. The performance of such algorithms depends on several factors, including the search direction relative to the ultrasound beam axis and whether they are applied to RF or detected signals. Correlation algorithms are computationally complex and therefore slow, but much simpler algorithms[61] based on absolute difference techniques have been shown to work adequately and have the potential to be implemented in real-time.

Given the developments in this field, it seems likely that before long, color-flow systems will provide the option of measuring the magnitude and direction of the velocity vectors in at least some of the field of view. A further development would be to extend either or both of the techniques described here to three dimensions, and although several practical problems must be overcome before this becomes possible, this too seems an inevitable step.

Display Techniques

To make the best use of the large amount of information that can now be obtained from CFI systems, better display techniques will be required in the future. This will be particularly so if vector fields are to be displayed. So far it appears that little has been published on this subject, although some interesting work has been carried out on methods of presenting vectorial velocity data by means of color coding.[61–63]

CONCLUSIONS

Although CFI has achieved a high level of clinical acceptance in what has so far been a relatively short life, it is still at an early stage in its development and considerable improvements and innovations can be anticipated during the next few years. Among these almost certainly will be new transducer technologies, better methods for rejecting "fixed target" echoes, new frequency estimation algorithms, more effective methods for overcoming aliasing limitations, vector Doppler systems that alleviate some of the problems associated with measuring only a single component of velocity, and display techniques that make better use of all the information that current and future CFI systems are and will be capable of providing.

CFI has revolutionized ultrasound in general and Doppler in particular, and many more exciting technical and clinical developments can be expected of it in the near future.

REFERENCES

1. Hokanson DE, Mozersky DJ, Sumner DS, Strandness DE: Ultrasonic arteriography: a new approach to arterial visualisation. Biomed Eng 6:420, 1971
2. Mozersky DJ, Hokanson DE, Baker DW et al: Ultrasonic arteriography. Arch Surg 103: 663, 1971
3. Spencer MP, Reid JM, Davis DL, Paulson PS: Cervical carotid imaging with a continuous-wave Doppler flowmeter. Stroke 5:145, 1974
4. Fish PJ: Multichannel, direction-resolving Doppler angiography. p. 153. In Kazner E, de Vlieger M, Muller HR, McCready VR (eds): Ultrasonics in Medicine. Excerpta Medica, Amsterdam, 1975
5. Curry GR, White DN: Colour coded ultrasonic differential velocity arterial scanner (echoflow). Ultrasound Med Biol 4:27, 1977
6. Brandestini M: Topoflow—a digital full range Doppler velocity meter. IEEE Trans Sonics Ultrason 25:287, 1978
7. Eyer MK, Brandestini MA, Phillips DJ, Baker DW: Color digital echo/Doppler image presentation. Ultrasound Med Biol 7: 21, 1981
8. Namekawa K, Kasai C, Tsukamoto M, Koyano A: Imaging of blood flow using autocorrelation. Ultrasound Med Biol 8:138, 1982
9. Namekawa K, Kasai C, Tsukamoto M, Koyano A: Realtime bloodflow imaging system utilizing auto-correlation techniques. p. 203. In Lerski RA, Morley P (eds): Ultrasound '82. Pergamon Press, New York, 1982
10. Kasai C, Namekawa K, Koyano A, Omoto R: Real-time two-dimensional blood flow imaging using an autocorrelation technique. IEEE Trans Sonics Ultrason 32:458, 1985
11. Bonnefous O, Pesque P, Bernard X: A new velocity estimator for color flow mapping. Proc IEEE Ultrason Symp 855, 1986
12. Bonnefous O, Pesque P: Time domain formulation of pulse-Doppler ultrasound and blood velocity estimation by cross correlation. Ultrason Imaging 8:73, 1986
13. Angelsen BAJ: On the design of 2D flow imaging systems. Meeting of the University of Trondheim Biomedical Research Group. Trondheim, Norway, 1986
14. Nowicki A, Reid JM: An infinite gate pulse Doppler. Ultrasound Med Biol 7:41, 1981

15. Shrader WW: MTI radar. p. 17.1. In Skolnik MI (ed): Radar Handbook. McGraw-Hill, New York, 1970

16. Fletcher RH, Burlage DW: An initialization technique for improved MTI performance in phased array radars. IEEE Proc 60:1551, 1972

17. Willemetz JC, Nowicki A, Meister JJ et al: Bias and variance in the estimate of the Doppler frequency induced by a wall motion filter. Ultrason Imaging 11:215, 1989

18. Evans DH, McDicken WN, Skidmore R, Woodcock JP: Doppler Ultrasound: Physics, Instrumentation, and Clinical Applications. Wiley, Chichester, 1989

19. Kitney RI, Giddens DP: Linear estimation of blood flow waveforms measured by Doppler ultrasound. MEDINFO 86:672, 1986

20. Kaluzynski K: Analysis of application possibilities of autoregressive modelling to Doppler blood flood signal spectral analysis. Med Biol Eng Comput 25:373, 1987

21. Schlindwein FS, Evans DH: A real-time autoregressive spectrum analyzer for Doppler ultrasound signals. Ultrasound Med Biol 15: 263, 1989

22. Gerzberg L, Meindl JD: Power-spectrum centroid detection for Doppler systems applications. Ultrason Imaging 2:236, 1980

23. Kristoffersen K, Angelsen BAJ: A comparison between mean frequency estimators for multigated Doppler systems with serial signal processing. IEEE Trans Biomed Eng 32:645, 1985

24. van Leeuwen GH, Hoeks APG, Reneman RS: Simulation of real-time frequency estimators for pulsed Doppler systems. Ultrason Imaging 8:252, 1986

25. Nowicki A, Reid J, Pedersen PC et al: On the behavior of instantaneous frequency estimators implemented on Doppler flow imagers. Ultrasound Med Biol 16:511, 1990

26. Lunt MJ: Accuracy and limitations of the ultrasonic Doppler blood velocimeter and zero crossing detector. Ultrasound Med Biol 2:1, 1975

27. Hoeks APG, Reneman RS, Peronneau PA: A multigate pulsed Doppler system with serial data processing. IEEE Trans Sonics Ultrason 28:242, 1981

28. Hoeks APG, Peeters HHPM, Ruissen CJ, Reneman RS: A novel frequency estimator for sampled Doppler signals. IEEE Trans Biomed Eng 31:212, 1984

29. Grandchamp PA: A novel pulsed directional Doppler velocimeter: the phase detection profilometer. p. 137. In Kazner E, de Vlieger M, Muller HR, McCready VR (eds): Ultrasonics in Medicine. Excerpta Medica, Amsterdam, 1975

30. Brandestini M: Application of the phase detection principle in a transcutaneous velocity profile meter. p. 144. In Kazner E, de Vlieger M, Muller HR, McCready VR (eds): Ultrasonics in Medicine. Excerpta Medica, Amsterdam, 1975

31. Barber WD, Eberhard JW, Karr SG: A new time domain technique for velocity measurements using Doppler ultrasound. IEEE Trans Biomed Eng 32:213, 1985

32. Brandestini MA, Forster FK: Blood flow imaging using a discrete-time frequency meter. Proc IEEE Ultrason Symp 3, 1978

33. Gill RW: Performance of the mean frequency Doppler modulator. Ultrasound Med Biol 5: 237, 1979

34. Foster SG, Embree PM, O'Brien WD: Flow velocity profile via time-domain correlation: error analysis and computer simulation. IEEE Trans Ultrason Ferroelec Freq Contr 37:162, 1990

35. Embree PM, O'Brien WD: Volumetric blood flow via time-domain correlation: experimental verification. IEEE Trans Ultrason Ferroelec Freq Contr 37:176, 1990

36. Newhouse VL, Ehrenwald AR, Johnson GF: The effect of Rayleigh scattering and frequency dependent absoption on the output spectrum of Doppler blood flowmeters. p. 1181. In White D, Brown RE (eds): Ultrasound in Medicine. Plenum Press, New York, 1977

37. Holland SK, Orphanoudakis SC, Jaffe CC: Frequency-dependent attenuation effects in pulsed Doppler ultrasound: experimental results. IEEE Trans Biomed Eng 31:626, 1984

38. Round WH, Bates RHT: Modification of spectra of pulses from ultrasonic transducers by scatterers in non-attenuating and in attenuating media. Ultrason Imaging 9:18, 1987

39. Light LH: Effect of selective tissue attenuation on pulsed Doppler frequency. Ultrasound Med Biol 16:317, 1990

40. Leeman S, Thomas N, Healey AJ, Williams RE: Problems in pulsed Doppler. p. 220. In: Proceedings of Eurodop '92. BMUS, London, 1992

41. de Jong PGM, Arts T, Hoeks APG, Reneman RS: Determination of tissue motion velocity by correlation interpolation of pulsed ultrasonic echo signals. Ultrason Imaging 12:84, 1990

42. Kristoffersen K, Angelsen BAJ: A time-shared ultrasound Doppler measurement and 2-D imaging system. IEEE Trans Biomed Eng 35:285, 1988

43. Takeuchi Y: Color coded Doppler scans. Ultrasound Med Biol 13:151, 1987

44. Loupas T, McDicken WN: Low-order complex AR models for mean and maximum frequency estimation in the context of Doppler color flow mapping. IEEE Trans Ultrason Ferroelec Freq Contr 37:590, 1990

45. Ahn YB, Park SB: Estimation of mean frequency and variance of ultrasonic Doppler signal by using second-order autoregressive model. IEEE Trans Ultrason Ferroelec Freq Contr 38:172, 1991

46. Ferrara KW, Algazi VR: A new wideband spread target maximum likelihood estimator for blood velocity estimation—Part I: Theory. IEEE Trans Ultrason Ferroelec Freq Contr 38:1, 1991

47. Ferrara KW, Algazi VR: A new wideband spread target maximum likelihood estimator for blood velocity estimation—Part II: Evaluation of estimators with experimental data. IEEE Trans Ultrason Ferroelec Freq Contr 38:17, 1991

48. Jerri AJ: The Shannon sampling theorem—its various extensions and applications: a tutorial review. Proc IEEE 65:1565, 1977

49. Nyquist H: Certain topics in telegraph transmission theory. AIEE Trans 47:617, 1928

50. Bendick PJ, Newhouse VL: Ultrasonic random-signal flow measurement system. J Acoust Soc Am 56:860, 1974

51. Cathignol DJ, Fourcade C, Chapelon J-Y: Transcutaneous blood flow measurements using pseudorandom noise Doppler system. IEEE Trans Biomed Eng 27:30, 1980

52. Hartley CJ: Resolution of frequency aliases in ultrasonic pulsed Doppler velocimeters. IEEE Trans Sonics Ultrason 28:69, 1981

53. Baek KR, Bae MH, Park SB: A new aliasing extension method for ultrasonic 2-dimensional pulsed Doppler systems. Ultrason Imaging 11:233, 1989

54. Fehr R, Dousse B, Grossniklaus B: New advances in colour flow mapping: quantitative velocity measurement beyond the Nyquist limit. Br J Radiol 64:651, 1991

55. Fan P, Nanda NC, Cooper JW: Color Doppler assessment of high flow velocities using a new technology: in-vitro and clinical studies. Echocardiography 7:763, 1990

56. Daigle RE, Miller CW, Histand MB: Nontraumatic aortic blood flow sensing by use of an ultrasonic esophageal probe. J Appl Physiol 38:1153, 1975

57. Farthing S, Peronneau P: Flow in the thoracic aorta. Cardiovasc Res 13:607, 1979

58. Overbeck JR, Beach KW, Strandness DE: Vector Doppler: accurate measurement of blood velocity in two dimensions. Ultrasound Med Biol 18:19, 1992

59. Trahey GE, Hubbard SM, von Ramm OT: Angle independent ultrasonic blood flow detection by frame-to-frame correlation of B-mode images. Ultrasonics 26:271, 1988

60. Ramamurthy BS, Trahey GE: Potential and limitations of angle-independent flow detection algorithms using radio-frequency and detected echo signals. Ultrason Imaging 13:252, 1991

61. Bohs LN, Trahey GE: A novel method for angle independent ultrasonic imaging of blood flow and tissue motion. IEEE Trans Biomed Eng 38:280, 1991

62. Charles RD: Viewing velocity in flow fields. ASME Mech Eng 111:64, 1989

63. Vera N, Steinman DA, Ethier CR et al: Visualization of complex flow fields, with application to the interpretation of color flow Doppler images. Ultrasound Med Biol 18:1, 1992

9

Ultimate Limits in Ultrasound Image Resolution

Rachel A. Harris
Peter N. T. Wells

Three aspects of resolution are relevant to ultrasound imaging: spatial resolution, contrast resolution, and temporal resolution. Spatial resolution describes the ability of an imaging system to produce separately distinguishable registrations in the displayed image of closely positioned structures within the patient. Contrast resolution is a measure of the ability to produce separately distinguishable differences in the brightness of the registrations in the displayed image of structures with slightly different echogenicities within the patient. Temporal resolution is the ability of the imaging system to display changes with time in anatomic relationships within the patient.

RESOLUTION

Spatial Resolution

Spatial resolution can be defined as the reciprocal of the minimum distance between two very small reflectors (i.e., point targets)

within the patient (i.e., the object) at which separate registrations can just be detected in the image. An alternative definition, equivalent in principle and usually much more convenient in practice, is that the spatial resolution is equal to the reciprocal of the distance that appears in the image to correspond to a point target in the object. This definition avoids the need for a complicated phantom for the measurement of resolution[1]; moreover, it introduces the concept of the *sample volume* (or *resolution cell*), which is discussed later. It also avoids the problem of interference between the echo signals from separate targets that occurs when the signals begin to overlap so that the detected echo amplitude fluctuates according to the individual phases.

Strict usage of the term *resolution* relates to the reciprocal of the minimum distance between separately identifiable targets; its units are, for example, "per centimeter." Note that the smaller the distance, the higher the numeric value of the resolution. The term is also commonly used to identify the actual distance, rather than its reciprocal. Thus, for example, a system able to resolve 10 separate targets per centimeter may be said to have a resolution of 1 mm.

An ultrasound imaging system is likely to have several different values of spatial resolution. Thus, the beamwidth is typically five times greater than the length of the ultrasound pulse.[2] Moreover, the beam may not be circular in cross-section. A fairly complete

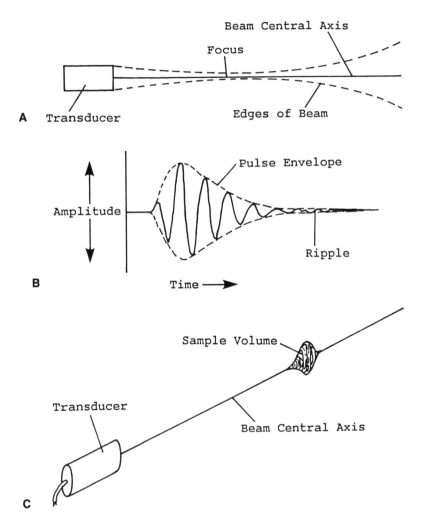

Fig. 9-1 Beam geometry, pulse length, and sample volume. **(A)** Edges of the beam are determined by size of transducer in relation to wavelength, and focusing arrangements. **(B)** Pulse length is determined by the envelope of the ultrasound pulse. **(C)** Sample volume is the three-dimensional "resolution cell"; it is shaped like a pointed teardrop and travels along central axis of the beam.

description of the resolution can be provided by specifying the dimensions of the volume of tissue occupied by the ultrasound pulse, from which backscattered echoes may be detected. This is called the *sample volume*[2] (Fig. 9-1). At any particular dynamic range (discussed later), the length of the sample volume, equivalent to the range resolution, depends on the length of the ultrasound pulse; its width within the scan plane determines the resolution in azimuth, whereas the thickness of the scan plane is equivalent to the resolution in elevation. A further complication is that the spatial resolution also is likely to have different values at different positions within the scan.

Contrast Resolution

Whether a signal can be detected is determined partly by the contrast resolution of the imaging system. The contrast resolution can be defined as the minimum difference in the amplitudes of two signals that can be detected as, for example, an edge or a disk of specified size in the image. Like the spatial resolution, the value of the contrast resolution generally depends on the position within the scan plane. This subject is discussed in detail in Chapter 1.

Human observers are limited in their ability to perceive visual information.[3] For example, for image signals subtending angles smaller than 1 mrad at the eye, the unsharpness of the eye plays an important role in detectability. The definitions of both spatial and contrast resolutions involve the concept of signal detectability, and thus they are inextricably linked.[4] In an image of two closely positioned targets, the presence of separately distinguishable registrations depends partly on the adjustment of the contrast of the display. Reducing the dynamic range of the display so that signals with nearly equal amplitudes produce very different brightnesses increases the likelihood of detecting the two

targets but reduces the accuracy of the measurement of the distance between them.[2]

Temporal Resolution

In two-dimensional imaging, the temporal resolution is limited by the image frame rate. (In one-spatial-dimensional scanning such as M-mode ultrasound time-position recording, the temporal resolution is limited by the pulse repetition rate.) Two-dimensional ultrasound images are made up of some number of individual scan lines arranged, for example, in sector or rectangular format. Ultimately, the maximum frame rate (i.e., the temporal resolution) depends on the depth of penetration and the speed of ultrasound. Similar considerations apply to three-dimensional imaging.

TISSUE CHARACTERISTICS AFFECTING RESOLUTION

Speed

The speed of ultrasound in soft tissues[5] is about 1,500 m/s and can be considered to be independent of the frequency. The usual approach to the design of an imaging system begins with the specification of the required maximum depth of penetration into the patient. For an abdominal scanner, for example, this depth typically might be 15 cm. This corresponds to a go-and-return time delay of 200 μs between the transmission of a pulse and the reception of an echo from the deepest structure. This go-and-return time delay determines the maximum pulse repetition rate that can be used, because the echo from the deepest structure has to be received before another pulse can be transmitted if ambiguity is to be avoided. In the present example, the corresponding maximum pulse repetition rate is 5,000 pulses per second. In a two-dimensional imaging system, the image frame rate is equal to the pulse repetition rate divided by the number of lines per frame. Thus, with 5,000 pulses per second, there could be 100 lines per frame at 50 frames per second, and so on.

The situation is more complicated with color-flow imaging. In color-flow imaging systems using the Doppler effect and autocorrelation detection,[6] at least three ultrasound pulses need to be transmitted in any particular direction to obtain a measurement of phase change. This alone is insufficient to give an estimate of target velocity, and it is usual for at least eight pulses to be needed for this. Thus, the image frame rate is likely to have to be at least eight times slower than that for two-dimensional gray-scale imaging for the same number of lines in the image. System designers usually compromise by having a sparser line density; this is discussed in more detail later. As in any Doppler system, the Nyquist sampling theorem[2] applies. The pulse repetition rate has to be at least twice the maximum Doppler shift frequency if ambiguity is to be avoided. Moreover, the maximum image frame rate is ultimately limited by the minimum velocity that it is desired to detect.[2] This is because sufficient pulse-echo samples have to be obtained in every direction within the scan; for each direction, it is the measurement of the lowest Doppler shift frequency that takes the longest time. Color-flow imaging based on time domain processing[7] is, in principle, free from these limitations. The only constraint is that the moving ensemble (explained later) has to remain in the ultrasound beam for long enough for its motion to be estimated from pulse-echo measurements of ensemble position.

Interest is growing in the acquisition and display of three-dimensional ultrasound images.[8] Such images can be considered to be made up of some number of contiguous two-dimensional ultrasound scans. As already explained, a certain time is required for the collection of each two-dimensional scan plane. The scanning time for the three-dimensional volume depends on the number of contiguous planes necessary to give acceptably close spacing; this spacing is unlikely to be much different from the line spacing within any two-dimensional scan plane.

Different tissues may have different ultrasound propagation speeds. Published data reveal a wide range of variation[5] from 1,412 m/s in fat to 1,629 m/s in muscle. The speed is even higher in cartilage and hard tissues. Ultrasound scanners are calibrated at an "average" value of speed, and so the calculation of distance within the patient may be in error when based on measurements taken from images. The spatial distortion of images is usually negligible, however, because it does not significantly affect an observer's ability to interpret anatomic relationships.

Attenuation

The attenuation of ultrasound in soft tissues is about 0.5 dB/cm at a frequency of 1 MHz, and it increases approximately in proportion to the frequency.[5] In principle, in an ultrasound imaging system the spatial resolution increases as the wavelength of the ultrasound becomes shorter (Fig. 9-2). Because the wavelength is inversely proportional to the frequency, system designers generally seek to use the maximum possible ultrasound frequency. The fundamental requirement is that the weakest significant echo from the maximum depth of penetration in the patient must have sufficient amplitude to be detectable. A signal can be detected only if its amplitude exceeds that of the noise of the system. *Noise* is the technical term used to describe artifactual signals that tend to mask the required information, such as the echoes from structures within the patient. Two kinds of noise are relevant to ultrasound imaging: biologic noise (e.g., speckle, which is discussed later); and electric noise, which arises within the receiver and which, for a

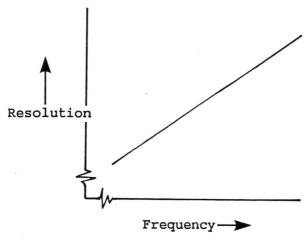

Fig. 9-2 Relationship between spatial resolution and ultrasound frequency. As frequency is increased, the wavelength becomes shorter.

given frequency bandwidth, is determined by fundamental physical phenomena over which the system designer has little or no control.

In contemporary ultrasound equipment, the maximum penetration at which detectable signals can be obtained is equal to about 400 wavelengths.[9] Expressed in this way, the penetration is independent of the frequency, but the wavelength depends on the frequency. Thus, for example, a penetration of 15 cm into the patient corresponds to 400 wavelengths at a frequency of 4 MHz.

Scattering

An ultrasound wave is scattered when it travels through tissue.[2] The geometry of the scattering depends on the dimensions of the structures of the tissue in relation to the ultrasound wavelength. At one extreme, the scattering surface may be smooth and extensive (e.g., the interface between the liver and the diaphragm). In this case, the ultrasound beam is reflected in a specular fashion so that the angle of reflection is equal to the angle of incidence. At the other extreme, the scatterer may be tiny in relation to the wavelength (this is the situation with a single red blood cell at low megahertz frequencies[2]). The incident ultrasound wave is then scattered uniformly in all directions (i.e., scattering is isotropic), and the amplitude of the scattered radiation is proportional to the fourth power of the frequency. Usually, soft tissues can be considered to be made up of many small scatterers. Although each of these scatterers behaves more or less isotropically, the backscattered signal that is detected arises from ensembles of these scatterers. The amplitude of the detected signal depends on the spatial distribution of the scatterers making up the ensemble within the sample volume of the imaging system. Each of the separately radiated spherical wavelets arising from the individual scatterers within the ensemble interferes at the receiving transducer in a way that depends on the individual phases and amplitudes. The result of this interference is highly dependent on the precise positions of the ensembles, and the effect is to produce a detected echo amplitude that fluctuates markedly with small changes in position.[10] The spatial fluctuation appears as a mottle pattern in the image, known as speckle; an analogous and familiar phenomenon occurs in optics with laser light.

The amplitude of the backscattered wave, in a macroscopic way, also depends on the relative effects of attenuation in overlying tissues and scattering power within the sample volume. As already explained, the scattering from blood, for example, depends on the fourth power of the frequency; but the attenuation in overlying tissue increases in proportion to the frequency. Consequently, at any particular penetration, the detected backscattered amplitude has a maximum value at some particular value of frequency. A practical example of this effect occurs in duplex scanning, where a higher frequency usually is used for imaging (for which high spatial resolution is required) than the frequency that gives the maximum amplitude Doppler signal for flow measurement.

Inhomogeneity

Ultrasound beams become distorted as they travel through biologic tissues. In laboratory experiments, the distortion may seem to be alarming; for example, in traveling through a human calf, the unfocused beam of a 20-mm-diameter 1.5-MHz transducer may have a displacement that has been typically measured[11] to be about 20 mm (Fig. 9-3). This beam distortion arises primarily because of differences in the propagation speeds in the different tissues through which the beam is passing. The phenomenon is known as *phase aberration*.

Because nothing can be done to eliminate phase aberration within the tissue, an ideal ultrasound imaging system would incorporate a method of correcting for its effect. One way in which this could be performed would involve the use of a two-dimensional transducer array consisting of a matrix of small transducer elements, each with its own electronic signal processing path.[8] Because of tissue inhomogeneity, the echoes detected by each element from a point target within the patient would arrive at different times (in addition to the time differences caused by path

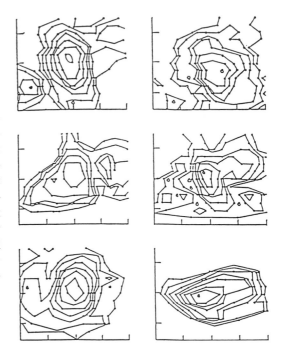

Fig. 9-3 Pulse-echo beam plots of isoecho amplitude contours for calves of six limbs. Plots were made using a 20-mm-diameter steel ball target; range was 150 mm, and the 20-mm-diameter unfocused transducer generated at a frequency of 1.5 MHz. Contour intervals are 5 dB, and grid spacing is 10 mm. (Courtesy of M. Halliwell.)

length differences) at each element in the array. The beam could be accurately focused on the point target by introducing the appropriate compensating time delay in each signal path. Because of the complexity of the system and the practical inability to realize the point target reference requirement, the technique has not been tested so far outside one or two advanced laboratories. As an alternative to the point target, the speckle brightness may be maximized to optimize the phase aberration correction.[12]

Although phase aberration is one of the mechanisms that ultimately limits the achievable ultrasound imaging resolution, it is worth pointing out that the degrading effect of the phenomenon is not as bad as might be expected from a simple interpretation of the beam distortion measured experimentally in the laboratory for one-way transmission through tissue, as mentioned earlier. This is because, in pulse-echo ultrasound imaging, the backscattered ultrasound retraces the beam path through the intervening tissue. Any phase aberration introduced on the outward journey is corrected, to a first approximation, on the return journey. System designers usually use focused ultrasound beams, as discussed later, and the improvement in resolution that results from focusing does increase as the size of the aperture increases but only to a limited extent.[13] This is because the self-compensating effect of intervening tissue on phase aberration ultimately becomes less effective as greater volumes of tissue are involved.

Nonlinearity

Increasing the intensity of an ultrasound wave increases the nonlinearity of its propagation.[14] As the distance from the transducer increases, an initial sine wave is converted into a sawtooth, which then reverts to a sine wave as the amplitude is reduced by attenuation. This can be explained in physical terms by understanding that the propagation speed is dependent on the density of the medium through which the wave is traveling. The density changes with the pressure of the wave, being greater during positive-ongoing pressure excursions. In the sawtooth region, the consequent increase in attenuation (resulting from the presence of higher-frequency components) may lead to an excess attenuation by a factor of up to about 2.[14] Despite this seemingly alarming effect, however, there does not seem to be any noticeable change in image appearances.[15]

Obviously, the intensity of ultrasound used in imaging should be kept as low as possible because of safety considerations. This is discussed in the next section. Nevertheless, the generation of higher-frequency components by tissue nonlinearity can change the shape of the ultrasound beam significantly at high intensities (Fig. 9-4). The side lobes of the beam become more marked and the central lobe becomes broader as the intensity is increased.[16]

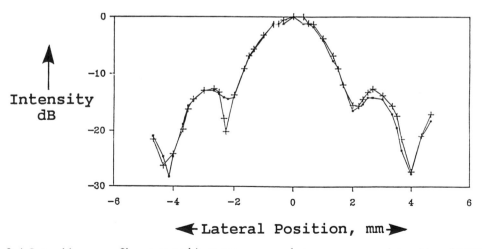

Fig. 9-4 Lateral beam profiles measured in water, measured at average source intensities of 0.087 W/cm^2 (——) and 2.24 W/cm^2 (—+—). Long pulses (100 cycles) were produced by a 2.25-MHz transducer with a diameter of 25 mm. Beam profile intensities are normalized to 0 dB in central axis. (Data from Reilly and Parker.[16])

SAFETY CONSIDERATIONS AFFECTING RESOLUTION

The prudent use of ultrasound diagnosis depends on an appropriate balance between cost and benefit. In this context, the cost includes the deficit caused by the hypothetical damage, including radiation damage to the patient, the public, and the staff, done by the test.[17] So far, qualitative methods of sufficient refinement to estimate this deficit have not been developed yet. Meanwhile, it is reasonable for equipment designers and users to apply the "as low as reasonably achievable" (ALARA) principle, although regulators of medical practice may seek to apply more rigorous controls. This is not the place to discuss their sometimes seemingly arbitrary nature.

If the attenuation is assumed to be proportional to the ultrasound frequency, it can be calculated that doubling the ultrasound intensity results in an increase in frequency (for the same echo amplitude at a given penetration) corresponding to a resolution improvement of about 5 percent.[18] This calculation neglects the effects of changes in scattering and nonlinearity. Thus, increasing the intensity is not an attractive way of increasing the ultrasound imaging resolution, because only a small improvement could arise from what certainly would be a worrisome potential decrease in safety.

OPTIMIZATION OF RESOLUTION

Beam Focusing

The field of an ultrasound transducer has a near-zone and a far-zone. In the near-zone, the field is roughly cylindrical but the beam diverges in the far-zone. The length of the near-zone increases with the diameter of the transducer and the ultrasound frequency. Within the near-zone, the beam can be focused, and this is usually done to improve spatial resolution. With a very large aperture and a homogeneous medium, very tight focusing can be achieved. (For example, in the acoustic microscope, the diameter of the focus can approach the theoretic limit set by the wavelength.[19]) In traditional ultrasound scanning, lens focusing does result in a very useful improvement in resolution, although only over a restricted depth of focus. The designer has to compromise between the resolution improvement at the focus and the depth of penetration over which imaging has to be carried out.

With an annular array, the beam can be focused at any chosen depth within the patient by appropriate choice of the time delays for the excitation of each transducer element. On reception, the time delays can be swept with time so that the beam is dynamically focused continuously to coincide with the instantaneous position of the echo-producing targets lying along the beam axis. Consequently, excellent spatial resolution can be obtained over a substantial depth range[20] by means of a mechanically scanned annular array transducer.

In scanners in which a one-dimensional array consisting of narrow strip transducers is used for two-dimensional imaging, fixed focusing can be applied on transmission and dynamic focusing on reception. This benefit is limited, however, to azimuthal resolution within the scan plane; it cannot be used to control the thickness of the scan (i.e., the resolution in elevation).[21] The thickness of the scan is usually minimized by lens focusing, to which the constraints that have already been discussed apply. In the future, it is likely that two-dimensional arrays of the kind already mentioned in connection with phase aberration correction[8] will become widely available, and they will allow dynamic focusing equivalent to that currently obtainable with annular arrays to be applied at the same time as electronically controlled beam steering within three dimensions.

It has already been explained that spatial and contrast resolutions are linked inextricably in the perceived image. Another practical connection between spatial and contrast resolutions arises from the geometry of the ultrasound beam. An ultrasound transducer produces a beam that is not simply concentrated around the central axis but that also has subsidiary lobes (or skirts) that spread out at theoretically predictable amplitudes and angles from the central axis.[2] For a given diameter of transducer, the amplitudes of these side lobes increase with frequency but decrease in angular divergence. With an array, the side lobes can be minimized by electronic signal processing.[22] There is no way in which the ultrasound imaging instrument can distinguish between echoes detected by the main beam and by the side lobes; all detected echoes are displayed as if they originated along the central axis. Consequently, the contrast resolution may be degraded by artifactual echoes arising from the side lobes. Practically, this is most obvious when, for example, the main beam passes through an hypoechoic cyst while the associated side lobes pass through echogenic tissue so that echoes are registered within what should be the echo-free image of the cyst.

Speckle Reduction

The origin of ultrasound speckle has already been explained. The speckle pattern in the image does not have a one-to-one correspondence with echo-producing targets within the patient; rather, it is an artifact that depends on the characteristics of the imaging system. Although the speckle pattern is not a direct representation of the tissue,[10] individual ultrasound scanners (and types of scanners) do produce different speckle patterns for different tissues, and so diagnosticians learn to interpret images on the basis of their experience. Consequently, although physicists may argue in favor of speckle reduction (considering speckle to be an annoy-

ing artifact), clinicians have justifiable reservations about this.

Because ultrasound speckle arises as a result of fluctuations in scattering ensemble geometry, very small changes in position within the patient produce marked shifts in speckle patterns. Some ultrasound scanning equipment has the facility to average the most recently acquired sequence of ultrasound scans, and this results in speckle reduction.[10] Other methods of speckle reduction based on image filtration are actively being investigated in research laboratories.[23] The next stage in instrument design may incorporate optional speckle reduction, perhaps with the simultaneous display of conventional and speckle-reduced images, to aid the diagnostician. There may also turn out to be a role for computer-based quantitative image texture analysis,[24] because the human observer is not very good at identifying or distinguishing between different textures. For a fuller discussion of this subject, the reader is referred to Chapter 5.

Transducer Matching

The material from which ultrasound transducers are usually constructed is much denser and has a higher propagation speed than soft tissue. As a result, strong reflections occur between the surface of the transducer and the soft tissue unless a matching layer is used to improve the coupling efficiency. In its simplest form, the matching layer is a quarter of a wavelength in thickness and has a characteristic acoustic impedance (the product of the density and the propagation speed), which is the geometric mean of the characteristic impedances of the transducer and soft tissue.[25] To operate over a wide band of frequencies, however, matching layers consisting of several different thin sheets are used.[26]

Although the primary reason for using a matching layer is to minimize what is technically described as the insertion loss of the transducer, there is an additional benefit. If a matching layer is not used, the ultrasound pulse produced by a transducer is quite long, so that the sample volume and, consequently, the range resolution is rather poor—typically, five or six wavelengths. Moreover, the pulse is followed by ripple of annoyingly high amplitude[27] caused by reverberation within the transducer. The ripple is reflected by tissues and gives rise to echoes that reduce the contrast resolution in the same way that side lobe echoes reduce the contrast resolution, as has already been explained. The use of a well-designed matching layer, however, results in the production of a "clean" pulse relatively free from ripple.

Image Line Interpolation

The relationship between image frame rate and image line density has already been discussed. Usually, an adequate line density can be obtained with gray-scale real-time two-dimensional scanning even at rapid frame rates. This is seldom the case, however, in color-flow imaging or three-dimensional scanning. Although neither spatial nor contrast resolutions are quantitatively affected by line density, target detectability certainly is degraded in images with sparse lines. This is partly because the gaps between the lines are visually distracting and partly because the targets may be missed. The system designer can do nothing about missing targets, but the esthetic quality of the image can be greatly enhanced by interpolating synthetically generated image lines between the real information.[28] This approach is widely used in image processing in various fields. The observer should always remember that much of the image that is displayed (indeed, most of the image with some color-flow imaging systems) is a creation of the computer and not necessarily a representation of the patient. Naturally, manufacturers of ultra-

sound scanners are rather coy about the details of their individual stratagems.

Time Frequency Control

Attenuation determines the maximum usable frequency at the maximum depth of penetration, as has already been explained. There is no reason why the resolution needs to be determined by this frequency at depths of less than the maximum penetration. If a broadband ultrasound pulse is transmitted into the patient, the frequency to which the receiver is tuned can be swept downward with time (in a manner analogous to the use of swept gain to compensate for attenuation in traditional imaging machines).[29] An optimally designed swept frequency system eliminates the need for any swept gain control at all, because the receiver always operates at the maximum gain compatible with the detection of echo signals above the amplitude of the noise.

Other Possible Methods for Improving Resolution

SIGNAL AVERAGING

It has already been pointed out that the maximum frequency that can be used at any particular penetration in a traditional ultrasound imaging system is limited by attenuation. A higher frequency can be used if signal averaging is used[30] (Figs. 9-5 and 9-6). This depends on the fact that a repetitive signal buried in noise can be extracted by the simple addition of a sequential series of signals. Apart from changes caused by movement (either physiologic within the patient or caused by changes in the position of the scan plane), ultrasound imaging satisfies the repetitive signal condition. The reduction in the noise level is proportional to the square root of the number of images that are added. Signal averaging promises to allow the ul-

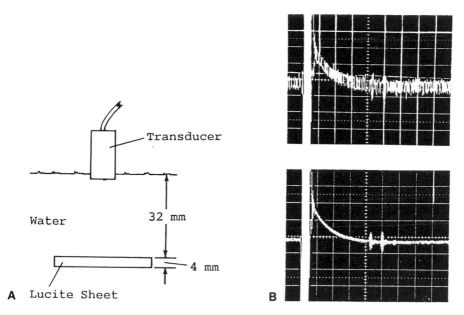

Fig. 9-5 Reduction of signal-to-noise ratio by signal averaging. **(A)** Experimental set-up. Ultrasound transducer operated at a frequency of 5 MHz. **(B)** Upper trace shows radio frequency signal from the transducer, with a single pulse-echo wavetrain. Lower trace is the result of averaging 10 pulse-echo wavetrains; echoes from surfaces of lucite sheet are clearly detectable above remaining noise, and the first multiple reflection echo is also visible.

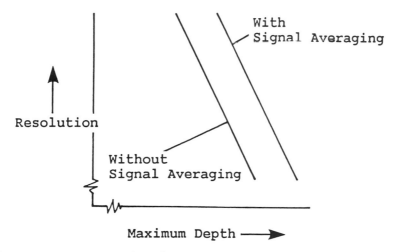

Fig. 9-6 Relationship between spatial resolution and maximum depth, without and with signal averaging. With signal averaging, a higher ultrasound frequency can be used while the signal-to-noise ratio (SNR) is maintained. Resolution increases with frequency, but as frequency is increased, maximum depth is reduced for a given value of SNR.

trasound frequency to be increased above the value set by biologic safety and nonlinearity considerations, with a consequent improvement in spatial resolution, but the extent to which this can be performed in any particular clinical situation remains to be determined.

Intuitively, a given quantity of energy should provide the same amount of information in diagnostic imaging, no matter how the energy is distributed in time. Thus, for a given total energy, there is no difference in principle between the use of a single high-amplitude pulse and the use of repetitive low-amplitude pulses with signal averaging. By spreading the delivery of energy over a longer time, signal averaging allows the same information to be collected but without the problems associated with nonlinearity and the anxiety about safety.

CONTRAST AGENTS

Potentially, contrast resolution can be increased by enhancing the differential scattering of different tissues. This can already be performed in some clinically useful situations by the use of ultrasound contrast agents such as microbubbles and particles.[31] Provided that the targeting scheme is selective (and it is useless if it is not), increasing the dose of contrast agent leads to an increase in contrast. In principle, the potential benefit is limited only by toxicity. For a fuller discussion of this subject, the reader is referred to Chapter 3.

DECONVOLUTION

In simple applications of ultrasound imaging (e.g., in nondestructive testing), the spatial resolution has been enhanced successfully by a process known as deconvolution,[32] in which the two-dimensional echo signal is fed through filters that compensate for the shape of the sample volume. The echo information obtained from biologic tissues is generally complicated, however, and deconvolution

has had only limited success in medical imaging.

SPATIAL MULTIPLEXING

In traditional ultrasound scanning, a single pulse of ultrasound is transmitted along a narrow beam in some particular direction and another pulse is not transmitted until all the echoes have been received. With some sacrifice in azimuthal resolution, however, it is possible, in principle, to transmit a rather broad ultrasound beam and simultaneously to receive separate echo wavetrains corresponding to different lines at slightly different angles within the broad transmitted beam. This spatial multiplexing process, called Explososcan,[33] allows the image frame rate to be increased (perhaps by a factor of 4), with a corresponding increase in temporal resolution. It has not been used yet in routine ultrasound scanning, but it is an attractive possibility, particularly to reduce the time necessary for three-dimensional imaging.

SYSTEM OPTIMIZATION

As an alternative to phase aberration correction with a two-dimensional array, as already discussed, a pragmatic and relatively easily realized approach to resolution improvement could be by system optimization.[30] In the proposed arrangements (Fig. 9-7), a two-dimensional real-time scan would be produced in the ordinary way. A region of interest, containing the structures to be displayed with enhanced resolution, would then be localized within the scan area. Generally, the region of interest would occupy an area with less width than the conventional scan and at less depth than the depth limit of the scan. By time sharing, the line density within the region of interest would be increased. Further improvement in spatial and contrast resolutions could be obtained at the expense of temporal resolution by reducing the image frame rate. Moreover, signal averaging would be applied to reduce the noise so that

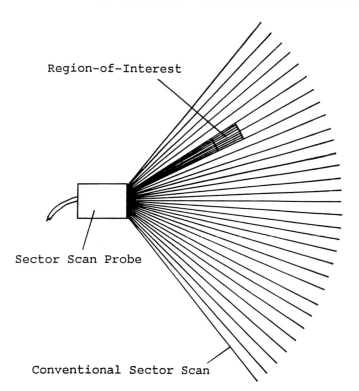

Fig. 9-7 In a system for resolution optimization, a sector scan probe is arranged to produce a conventional sector scan having a lower line density than that used to scan a small region of interest selected from within the scanned anatomy. The region of interest is likely to be situated at a smaller depth than maximum depth of the conventional scan.

the frequency could be optimized at the maximum usable range to provide the best possible resolution. The fundamental rationale for this approach is that a compact high-frequency beam is less likely to be affected adversely by tissue inhomogeneities than the beam of a conventional ultrasound scanner.

CONCLUSIONS

Although remarkable progress has already been made in ultrasound imaging, particularly during the last decade, there are still many opportunities for further improvements in image resolution. The development of the two-dimensional transducer array is perhaps the most challenging and likely in the longer term to be most widely applied. In the near future, however, techniques based on system optimization are more promising. Improved resolution would have immediate clinical benefits in most applications of ultrasound imaging.[30]

ACKNOWLEDGMENTS

This work was supported in part by a grant from the U.K. Medical Research Council. We are grateful to Mrs. J. R. Fish for excellent help with the preparation of the manuscript.

REFERENCES

1. Smith SW, Wager RF, Sandrik JM, Lopez H: Low contrast detectability and contrast/detail analysis in medical ultrasound. IEEE Trans Sonics Ultrason 30:164, 1983
2. Wells PNT: Biomedical Ultrasonics. Academic Press, London, 1977
3. Hill CR, Bamber JC, Crawford DC et al: What might echography learn from image science? Ultrasound Med Biol 17:559, 1991
4. Lopez H, Loew MH, Butler PF et al: A clinical evaluation of contrast-detail analysis for ultrasound images. Med Phys 17:48, 1990
5. Duck FA: Physical Properties of Tissue. Academic Press, London, 1990
6. Kasai C, Namekawa K, Konano A, Omoto R: Real-time two-dimensional blood flow imaging using an autocorrelation technique. IEEE Trans Sonics Ultrason 32:458, 1985
7. Bonnefous O, Pesque P: Time domain formulation of pulse-Doppler ultrasound and blood velocity estimation by cross-correlation. Ultrason Imaging 8:73, 1986
8. von Ramm OT, Smith SW, Pavy HG: High-speed ultrasound volumetric imaging system. IEEE Trans Ultrason Ferroelect Freq Contr 38:109, 1991
9. Wells PNT, Harris RA, Halliwell M: The envelope that tissue imposes on achievable ultrasonic imaging. J Ultrasound Med 11:433, 1992
10. Wells PNT, Halliwell M: Speckle in ultrasonic imaging. Ultrasonics 19:225, 1981
11. Mountford RA, Halliwell M: Physical sources of registration errors in pulse-echo ultrasonic systems. Med Biol Eng 11:33, 1973
12. Nock L, Trahey GE, Smith SW: Phase aberration correction in medical ultrasound using speckle brightness as a quality factor. J Acoust Soc Am 85:1819, 1989
13. Moshfeghi M, Waag RC: In vivo and in vitro ultrasound beam distortion measurements of a large aperture and a conventional aperture focused transducer. Ultrasound Med Biol 14:415, 1988
14. Starritt HC, Duck FA, Hawkins AJ, Humphrey VF: The development of harmonic distortion in pulsed finite-amplitude ultrasound passing through the liver. Phys Med Biol 31:1401, 1986
15. Parker KJ: Observation of nonlinear acoustic effects in B-scan imaging instrument. IEEE Trans Sonics Ultrason 32:4, 1985
16. Reilly CR, Parker KJ: Finite-amplitude effects on ultrasound beam patterns in attenuating media. J Acoust Soc Am 86:2339, 1989
17. Wells PNT: The prudent use of diagnostic ultrasound. Br J Radiol 59:1143, 1986
18. Kremkau FW: Clinical benefit of higher acoustic output levels. Ultrasound Med Biol 15, suppl. 1:69, 1989
19. Briggs A: An Introduction to Scanning Acoustic Microscopy. Oxford University Press, Oxford, 1985
20. O'Donnell M: A proposed annular array imaging system for contact B-scan applications. IEEE Trans Sonics Ultrason 29:331, 1982
21. Skolnick ML: Estimation of ultrasound beam width in the elevation (section thickness) plane. Radiology 180:286, 1991
22. Whittingham TA: Resolution and information limitations from transducer arrays. Phys Med Biol 36:1503, 1991
23. Bamber JC, Phelps JV: Real-time implementation of coherent speckle suppression in B-scan images. Ultrasonics 29:218, 1991
24. Oosterveld BJ, Thijssen JM, Hartman PC et al: Ultrasound attenuation and texture analysis of diffuse liver disease. Phys Med Biol 36:1039, 1991
25. Hunt JW, Arditi M, Foster FS: Ultrasound transducers for pulse-echo medical imaging. IEEE Trans Biomed Eng 30:453, 1983
26. Inoue T, Ohta M, Takahashi S: Design of ultrasonic transducers with multiple acoustic matching layers for medical application. IEEE Trans Ultrason Ferroelect Freq Contr 34:8, 1987
27. Hadjicostis AN, Hottinger CF, Rosen JJ, Wells PNT: Ultrasonic transducer materials for medical applications. Ferroelectrics 60:107, 1984
28. Lee MH, Kim JH, Park SB: Analysis of a scan conversion algorithm for real-time sector scanner. IEEE Trans Med Imaging 5:96, 1986
29. Claesson I, Salomonsson G: Frequency- and depth-dependent compensation of ultrasonic signals. IEEE Trans Ultrason Ferroelect Freq Contr 35:582, 1988

30. Harris RA, Follett DH, Halliwell M, Wells PNT: Ultimate limits in ultrasonic imaging resolution. Ultrasound Med Biol 17:547, 1991
31. de Jong N, Ten Cate FJ, Lancée CT, et al: Principles and recent developments in ultrasound contrast agents. Ultrasonics 29:324, 1991
32. Jeurens TJM, Somer JC, Smeets FAM, Hoeks APG: The practical significance of two-dimensional deconvolution in echography. Ultrason Imaging 9:106, 1987
33. Shuttuck DP, Weinshenker MD, Smith SW, von Ramm OT: Explososcan: a parallel processing technique for high speed ultrasound imaging with linear phased arrays. J Acoust Soc Am 75:1273, 1984

10

Blood Flow Quantitation:
Waveform Analysis, Volume Measurement, Tumor Flow, and the Role of Color Imaging

Christy K. Holland
Kenneth J. W. Taylor

There have been considerable improvements in the quality of ultrasound imaging during the past 20 years, culminating in the current generation of dynamic color-flow mapping devices. Quantitative techniques are relatively in their infancy, however, and the venerable fast Fourier transform, dating from the 1960s, remains the conventional signal processing technique. Parameters derived from the Doppler spectrum, such as the pulsatility indices, are relatively crude and imprecise ways to describe a given waveform. It seems likely that considerable intellectual effort will be expended during the next decade on developing more quantitative methods for accurate estimation of flow, imped-ance, and several other parameters relating to vessel elasticity and compliance. Such methodology might be applied clinically to provide more accurate estimates of volume flow and to enhance differentiation between neovascularity and flow in normal vessels and might aid in earlier recognition of vascular disease.

VOLUMETRIC FLOW QUANTITATION

Measurement of volumetric blood flow using traditional Doppler generally requires the determination of the Doppler angle, vessel size, and instantaneous spatial mean velocity. Instantaneous volume flow, $Q(t)$, formally is defined as the product of the spatial mean velocity, $\bar{v}(t)$, and the cross-sectional area of the vessel, $A(t)$, or

$$Q(t) = \bar{v}(t)A(t). \tag{1}$$

The time-averaged volume flow, $\overline{Q}$, is correlated with perfusion and is written

$$\overline{Q} = \frac{1}{T}\int_{t=0}^{t=T} \bar{v}(t)A(t)\, dt. \tag{2}$$

The period over which the time average is performed, T, is usually chosen to encompass several cardiac cycles. Several techniques for estimating the average vessel cross-sectional area and for determining the mean velocity have been explored. Each technique can potentially give accurate measurements of volume flow, but users must appreciate the large errors that may occur under certain circumstances. In the following sections, selected mean velocity and average cross-sectional area estimation techniques are reviewed and the associated clinical applications and practical limitations are characterized.

Uniform Insonification Method

A well-known Doppler method for the measurement of blood flow requires the ultrasound intensity and the distribution of scatterers to be uniform throughout the sample volume.[1] If this uniform insonification condition is met, the power spectral density of the Doppler signal represents the distribution of red cell velocities within the sample volume and the instantaneous mean velocity, $\bar{v}(t)$, may be calculated from the intensity-weighted, instantaneous mean Doppler shift, $\bar{f}_D(t)$ (the normalized first moment of the Doppler spectrum):

$$\bar{v}(t) = \frac{c\bar{f}_D(t)}{2\cos(\theta)f_o}, \tag{3}$$

where c is the speed of sound, θ is the angle of insonification, and f_o is the center fre-

quency of insonification. $\bar{f}_D(t)$ is given by

$$\bar{f}_D(t) = \frac{\int \Pi(f)f\, df}{\int \Pi(f)\, df} \tag{4}$$

where $\Pi(f)$ is the Doppler power spectrum. Thus, by substituting Equation 3 into Equation 2, the mean volumetric flow is given by

$$\overline{Q} = \frac{1}{T}\left(\frac{c}{2\cos(\theta)f_o}\right)\int_{t=0}^{t=T} \bar{f}_D(t)A(t)\, dt. \tag{5}$$

The simplest approach to estimating the cross-sectional area of the vessel is to measure the internal diameter, D, at a single point in the cardiac cycle and then to calculate the area on the assumption that the vessel is circular in cross section:

$$A = \frac{\pi}{4}D^2. \tag{6}$$

By assuming the area does not change significantly over time, the mean volumetric flow is given by

$$\overline{Q} = \frac{A}{T}\left(\frac{c}{2\cos(\theta)f_o}\right)\int_{t=0}^{t=T} \bar{f}_D(t)\, dt. \tag{7}$$

LIMITATIONS

Although this simple methodology works well in the in vitro situation, greater errors occur in vivo because of physiologic variables that lead to changes in the luminal area. The systolic increase in the arterial lumen may lead to unacceptable errors in the estimation of area because any errors in the diameter estimation are squared in the computation of area. These variations are even more marked in veins where large variations (approximately 20 percent) in area are associated with respiration. Important sources of error in this technique of determining the vessel area include incorrect assumptions about the vessel shape (the cross section may not be circular), changes in the vessel area over time caused by cardiac or respiration variation, the limited axial resolution of the pulse-echo system, and incorrect caliper settings. Even if the axial resolution is very good, the highest achievable accuracy is in the order of the wavelength of the imaging ultrasound (0.1 to 0.8 mm). Caliper setting errors arise because the speed of sound in blood (approximately 1,580 m/s) is greater than the speed of sound in soft tissue (approximately 1,540 m/s). Many duplex machines use the speed of sound in soft tissue to calibrate the calipers and thus may underestimate the vessel diameter by as much as 5 percent. Algorithms that evaluate Equation 5 directly by automatically tracking the changing position and size of the vessel lumen reduce this error significantly and are available on some machines.[2]

Nonuniform insonation of the blood vessel,[3] differential attenuation between soft tissue and blood,[4] intrinsic spectral broadening leading to frequency-dependent scattering,[5,6] high-pass filters designed to reject high-amplitude, low-frequency Doppler shifts (caused by vessel wall motion),[7] and a poor signal-to-noise ratio[8,9] all could affect the intensity-weighted mean frequency and thus the accuracy of the determination of the mean volumetric flow. Several factors can contribute to the lack of uniformity of the scattering of ultrasound across the vessel lumen including the distribution of ultrasound intensity within the sample volume, the geometry of the ultrasound beam relative to the vessel dimensions, and the uniformity of scatters (red blood cells) within the blood.[10,11]

The Doppler angle, θ, is usually estimated by rotating a dedicated cursor on the B–scan image to align it with the axis of the vessel. (The scan plane must be adjusted so that a reasonable length of the vessel is in the scan plane.) Flow is assumed to be parallel to the vessel wall. This assumption most certainly breaks down near branching vessels, anastomoses, and stenotic lesions where flow disturbance and helicity are most likely present. Because the cosine of θ determines the component of velocity measured, the error increases rapidly as θ approaches 90 degrees,

where the cosine function varies rapidly. The percentage of error in the flow measurement caused by a given error in the measurement of the angle ($\Delta\theta$ is 5 degrees, 10 degrees, 15 degrees, and 20 degrees, respectively) is plotted as a function of Doppler angle in Figure 10-1. Because of the large errors in the Doppler shift resulting from a small error in θ ($\Delta\theta$ is 10 degrees or less) for θ greater than 60 degrees, it is best to minimize θ whenever possible to reduce the error caused by angle uncertainty.

CLINICAL APPLICATIONS

Many authors have claimed to use the even insonation method in clinical trials, but few attempts have been made to produce an even intensity either by deliberately defocusing the beam or by using the far-field of a transducer. There is at least one notable exception to this generalization. In in vitro experiments, a correlation coefficient, r, of 0.99 has been achieved when ultrasound flowmetry was compared with electromagnetic flow rates.[1] Using the same method to measure flow in pig aorta, a correlation of 0.96 has been obtained when compared with electromagnetic flowmetry.[12] The technique has been applied in 118 normal pregnancies to measure the flow in the umbilical vein.[13] The flow rates increased during pregnancy up to 35 weeks and then decreased toward term. When expressed in flow per kilogram of fetal weight, a constant flow of 120 ml/min/kg was found, which decreased to 90 ml/min/kg toward term. When this method was applied to the study of flow in abnormal pregnancies, more than half had flow rates outside the normal range. Flow rates less than normal were seen in 10 of 11 fetuses affected by intrauterine growth retardation (IUGR). When the flow was reduced in proportion to the reduction in fetal weight, there was the greatest risk for an abnormal pregnancy outcome. Other fetuses had increased flow rates. In diabetes, increased flow was proportional to the increased fetal weight, whereas in *Rhe-*

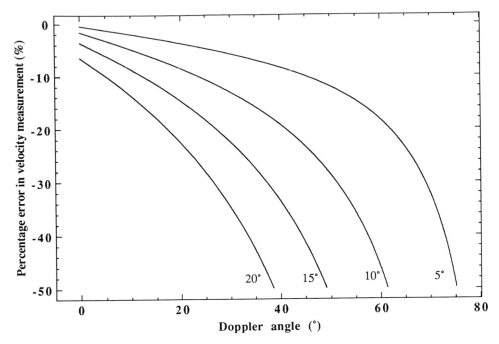

Fig. 10-1 Percentage error in velocity calculation caused by a given error; $\Delta\theta = 5$ degrees, 10 degrees, 15 degrees, and 20 degrees in the Doppler angle.

sus isoimmunization, antepartum hemorrhage, and pathologic placentae, there was an absolute increase in umbilical venous flow.

Calculated Mean Velocity Method

The relationship between the mean velocity calculated from volume flow capture and the angle-corrected maximum velocity has been determined experimentally from the Doppler frequency shift in an in vitro portal vein flow model over a range of physiologically relevant flow rates.[14] This empirical relationship was found to be

$$\bar{v}(t) = 0.57 v_{\max}. \tag{8}$$

Because the flow was continuous, it was assumed that the mean velocity did not vary significantly over time. This relationship has been applied in a study of portal blood flow in the normal Japanese population. To obtain the cross-sectional area of the portal vein, the

portal vein was imaged with a 5.0-MHz B-mode scanner to determine the diameter of the vessel from two angles, 90 degrees apart, and the formula for an ellipse was used.

The cross-sectional area of the portal vein was assumed to be independent of time as well, and thus the simple relationship for mean flow was used:

$$\overline{Q} = \bar{v}(t)A = (0.57 v_{\max})A. \tag{9}$$

The maximum velocity can be determined from the maximum Doppler shift, $f_{D\max}$, by substituting $v_{\max}$ using the well-known Doppler equation

$$\overline{Q} = 0.57 \left(\frac{c f_{D\max}}{2\cos(\theta) f_o} \right) A. \tag{10}$$

LIMITATIONS

Important sources of error in this technique of determining the vessel area include assumptions about the vessel shape (the cross section may not be elliptical, possibly because of disease), changes in the vessel area over time caused by cardiac or respiratory variation, the limited axial resolution of the pulse-echo system, and incorrect caliper settings. Similar considerations concerning inaccuracies in flow measurement caused by Doppler angle uncertainties apply to this calculated mean velocity method. Also, placement of the sample volume within the center of the lumen (the location assumed to contain the highest velocity) is crucial to the detection of the maximum Doppler shift, f_{Dmax}. Techniques for determining the maximum Doppler shift are generally more reliable than those for estimating the intensity-weighted mean Doppler shift because of their immunity to the effects of attenuation, noise, and high-pass filters.[15]

It is unlikely that arterial sites meet the appropriate criteria closely enough for this method to be of any value for estimating arterial flow. A variation of this method, however, which involves assuming a velocity profile, has been proposed.[16] In this technique, the mean velocity is approximated by

$$\bar{v}(t) = \kappa v_{max}, \tag{11}$$

where κ is a constant that depends on the time-averaged velocity profile. When the time-averaged velocity profile is flat or uniform across the lumen, κ is equal to 1. Similarly, when the time-averaged velocity profile is parabolic, corresponding to laminar flow, κ is 0.5. The time-averaged volumetric flow in this case is given by

$$\bar{Q} = \kappa \left(\frac{cf_{Dmax}}{2 \cos(\theta)f_o} \right) A. \tag{12}$$

CLINICAL APPLICATIONS

The technique based on Equation 8 has been applied widely in the measurement of portal venous flow, although the relationship between mean and maximum velocities is likely to be different in normals compared

with cirrhotics, who have a lower rate of flow. The inter- and intraobserver variations of this method of flow determination have been estimated.[17] This study provided information concerning reproducibility only and not accuracy of the method itself. In this study, two examiners made two measurements of portal venous flow on two consecutive mornings. Overall, the intraobserver variation, expressed as a coefficient of variation, was less than or equal to 14 ± 1 percent for one observer, but less satisfactory (less than or equal to 19 ± 3 percent) for the other. The interobserver variation (less than or equal to 20 ± 2 percent) also indicated considerable errors.

These results support only a limited use of this technique for the determination of rapid and large changes (greater than 100 percent) in portal hemodynamics within a short time. Because of its low precision, the technique is inappropriate for monitoring chronic changes in portal hemodynamics. This is unfortunate because there are many clinical situations in which a more accurate estimation of portal venous flow would be useful. For example, monitoring blood flow would be valuable in patients awaiting liver transplantation, where the detection of decreased flow could aid the prioritization of the waiting list for the procedure.

In further studies, the method has been used to measure flow in the superior mesenteric artery (SMA) and portal vein (PV) on 2 consecutive days in 12 cirrhotic patients and in 12 matched controls in response to a 355-kcal meal.[18] The flows were calculated from estimates of cross-sectional area and the mean velocity, which was calculated from the maximum velocity using the empirical correction factor of 0.57. Flows were estimated at 30-minute intervals from 0 to 150 minutes after the test meal. Baseline flows were similar in the cirrhotics and control patients. Maximal postprandial flow occurred at 30 minutes. The cirrhotic patients showed a blunted hyperemic response to food. Expressing PV flow as a percentage of the baseline value, the maximum postprandial flow was attained at 30 minutes at 189 ± 7 percent of the baseline value in controls and at 165 ± 6 percent in cirrhotics. Thus, the response in cirrhotics was blunted. In controls, the PV area significantly increased after a meal, whereas in the cirrhotics, the PV appeared to be almost maximally dilated at rest and increased flow was achieved only by increased velocity.

Flow in the SMA also showed similar baseline values for the two groups. After a meal, however, postprandial flow in normals peaked at 30 minutes at 144 ± 10 percent of the baseline value. In cirrhotics, these flow changes were subdued at 71 ± 32 percent of the baseline. Increased flow in the SMA was achieved by increased velocity without significant increase in area. This suggests that flow changes in the SMA can be monitored by peak velocity alone without the necessity of estimating volume flow with its recognized errors, especially those related to the measurement of area.

Attenuation-Compensated Method

A pulsed Doppler volumetric flowmeter that measures flow normal to an arbitrary, thin, uniform sample volume has been developed.[19] A two-element pulsed Doppler transducer interrogated two thin, concentric, sample volumes, assumed to be planes. Volume 1, as shown in Figure 10-2, encompasses the entire lumen of the vessel. The projection of the area of the lumen, $A(t)$, onto this sample plane is given by $A_{\text{proj}}(t)$. Note that

$$A(t) = A_{\text{proj}}(t)\cos(\theta) \qquad (13)$$

where θ is the Doppler angle. The second, smaller reference sample volume, volume 2, is chosen so that it lies completely within the vessel lumen. Using the notation in the original paper,[19] the total power in the two Doppler audio signals, $\Pi_1(t)$ and Π_2, produced by interrogating the flow with the two sample volumes is given by

$$\Pi_1(t) = T(z)\ \eta I_1(z)A_{\text{proj}}(t) \qquad (14a)$$

$$\Pi_2 = T(z)\eta I_2(z)A_2 \qquad (14b)$$

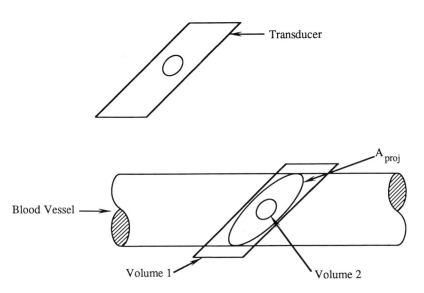

Fig. 10-2 Transducer configuration for the attenuation-compensated volumetric flowmeter.

where $T(z)$ is the round-trip transmission efficiency representing the effects of attenuation caused by transmission through tissue to a depth of z, η is the volumetric scattering coefficient of blood, and $I_1(z)$ and $I_2(z)$ indicate the sensitivities of transducer element 1 and transducer element 2, respectively, in the absence of the effects of attenuation. By substituting Equation 14a into Equation 13, an expression for the luminal area, $A(t)$, can be derived as a function of the total power in the first Doppler audio signal and parameters that are dependent on the measurement configuration and transducer characteristics only:

$$A(t) = \frac{\cos(\theta)\Pi_1(t)}{T(z)\eta I_1(z)}. \tag{15}$$

By substituting the expression for the luminal area, $A(t)$, from Equation 15 into Equation 5, the mean volumetric flow is given by

$$\overline{Q} = \frac{1}{T}\left(\frac{c}{2f_o}\right)\left(\frac{1}{T(z)\eta I_1(z)}\right)\int_{t=0}^{t=T}\overline{f}_D(t)\Pi_1(t)\,dt. \tag{16}$$

Note that this expression for flow is independent of the Doppler angle and that the precise vessel size need not be known to estimate $\overline{Q}$, as long as the vessel lumen lies entirely within the larger sample plane. The segment of vessel being interrogated, however, must be straight and have a uniform diameter. Variations in the lumen diameter during the cardiac cycle are thereby accommodated.

The power in the second Doppler audio signal, $\Pi_2(t)$, provides an indirect measurement of the product $T(z)\eta$, representing the combined effects of attenuation and target scattering efficiency. By solving for $T(z)\eta$ in Equation 14b and substituting the expression into Equation 16, $\overline{Q}$ is estimated by means of compensation for the combined effects of

scattering and attenuation (hence the name *attenuation-compensated volumetric flowmeter*):

$$\overline{Q} = \frac{1}{T}\left(\frac{c}{2f_o}\right)\left(\frac{A_2 I_2(z)}{\Pi_2 I_1(z)}\right)\int_{t=0}^{t=T}\overline{f}_D(t)\Pi_1(t)\,dt. \tag{17}$$

Note that f_o, A_2, $I_1(z)$, and $I_2(z)$ all must be assessed a priori for a particular transducer design.

LIMITATIONS

Several assumptions implicit in the development of this flowmeter must be examined to determine its validity in the clinical setting. The successful implementation of the flowmeter depends on uniform insonification of the entire vessel cross section, as well as the positioning of a narrow reference beam within the same cross section that lies entirely in the vessel lumen. A broad range of clinical applications further demands the adjustability of these beamwidths to facilitate selective insonification. Partial insonification of an outlying vessel may, for example, cause a large error in the estimate of flow through the vessel of interest. Also, any nonuniformity in the beam affects both the total power received and the mean Doppler shift, as already discussed. An annular array that promises to overcome many of these difficulties in the generation of a variable-width, uniform sector beam pattern has been developed.[20]

The practical requirements for the small sample volume are related to its function as a reference basis for detecting the effects of the scattering efficiency from blood and round-trip attenuation.[19] If the volume of blood within the second sample surface did not give rise to a representative measurement of the scattering efficiency and round-trip attenuation, this error would affect the mean volume flow estimation. For example, the "cell-free" zone observed near vessel walls[21] has been ignored, thus potentially limiting the clinical application of this technique to vessels larger than 5 mm. In addition, the effects of velocity or flow disturbance on the scattering efficiency are assumed to apply identically to all locations across the lumen. Poststenotic regions of flow, where recirculation close to the vessel wall and a central disturbed jet are present, potentially could pose a problem for this technique of flow estimation.

CLINICAL APPLICATIONS

Despite considerable interest in clinical applications of this technique, no results have yet been published.

SELECTED NORMALIZED INDICES FOR WAVEFORM SHAPE CHARACTERIZATION

The quantitation of volumetric flow is not the only method for extracting potentially clinically useful information from the Doppler waveform. The shape of the waveform may provide information about the state of the vascular bed as well. The shape of the Doppler waveform is a function of the mechanical parameters of the arterial system (e.g., vessel elasticity, distal impedance, and proximal lumen size). The recognition of certain pulsatile components of arterial Doppler waveforms may make it possible to detect proximal or distal disease. Several of the most commonly used feature extraction techniques are based on determining the ratio of the height or excursion of one portion of the waveform to that of another. The pulsatility index (PI), the resistive index (RI), and the systolic/diastolic ratio (S/D) are three such indices and are described in the following sections. The advantage of these simple ratios is that the Doppler waveform may be analyzed in either its frequency versus time or velocity versus time representation. Because the two representations differ only by a constant, the normalization process for each

index cancels the effect of such a constant. Hence these indices are independent of the Doppler angle, the frequency of insonification, and the speed of sound in the overlying tissue. None of these crude ratios, however, adequately describes all features of the Doppler waveform. For example, many different Doppler waveforms may give rise to the same index. Thus the original waveform cannot be reconstructed from any of these normalized indices.

Pulsatility Index

Originally it was attempted to extract information about the damping of the blood velocity waveform along an arterial pathway by defining a PI as the total energy in the velocity waveform divided by the energy in the instantaneous mean velocity waveform, time-averaged over the cardiac cycle.[22] A larger amount of damping evident in the arterial system would yield a smaller PI. Later, the definition of the PI was revised[23] to simplify its computation. The revised PI is defined as the peak-to-peak height of the Doppler waveform within one cardiac cycle, $f_{Dmax} - f_{Dmin}$, divided by the intensity-weighted mean Doppler shift $\bar{f}_D(t)$, time-averaged over the cardiac cycle, or

$$PI = \frac{f_{Dmax} - f_{Dmin}}{\dfrac{1}{T} \displaystyle\int_{t=0}^{t=T} \bar{f}_D(t)\, dt}, \qquad (18)$$

where T is the duration of the cardiac cycle. (Note that f_{Dmin} may be negative.) Because the time-averaged mean Doppler shift is difficult to compute and is subject to the errors already described, some duplex Doppler systems calculate a different PI, PI$'$, by dividing the peak-to-peak height of the Doppler waveform by the instantaneous peak Doppler shift, $f_{Dpk}(t)$, time-averaged over the cardiac cycle:

$$PI' = \frac{f_{Dmax} - f_{Dmin}}{\dfrac{1}{T} \displaystyle\int_{t=0}^{t=T} f_{Dpk}(t)\, dt} \qquad (19)$$

where again T is the duration of the cardiac cycle. (Some commercially available systems require the operator to trace the instantaneous peak Doppler shift envelope on the screen.) Care should be taken to ascertain whether PI or PI′ is computed by the particular Doppler system in use, and studies quoting PI values should state the particular definition of PI used to avoid confusion.

CLINICAL APPLICATIONS

There have been many clinical papers on the use of the PI, which originally was applied to ischemic disease of the lower extremity.[24] This index has been used to quantitate impedance of renal allografts in the early postoperative period.[24] An upper limit for a normal transplant was found to be a PI′ of 1.5. Higher values were found in acute rejection, particularly if a vascular component was present. Subsequent work showed many other rarer causes of increased impedance, which have been the subject of much discussion in the literature.[25]

The PI′ was determined off-line, using a digitizer. Subsequently, PI′ estimates have been included in the software of many commercial machines. Two different measures as outlined above, however, are used interchangeably in many machines so that this lack of universal agreement on this index adds much confusion to the literature and there seems to be little or no advantage in the use of the PI over the RI, which is easy to compute either on- or off-line.

Resistive Index

To avoid the problems associated with the estimation of the intensity-weighted mean Doppler shift, the RI, which is defined as the peak-to-peak height of the Doppler waveform within one cardiac cycle normalized by the systolic peak Doppler shift, was

devised[26]:

$$RI = \frac{f_{Dmax} - f_{Dmin}}{f_{Dmax}}. \qquad (20)$$

The advantage of the RI is that it is simple to calculate. An RI of 1 indicates no diastolic flow, which is often an important clinical observation. Reversal of flow during diastole (a negative f_{Dmin}) results in an RI greater than 1, indicating high peripheral impedance. Similarly, an RI less than 1 denotes flow into a low-impedance bed distally.

CLINICAL APPLICATIONS

The RI (or the resistance index) has been applied widely in many clinical examples in which loss of diastolic flow and reversal of flow are extremely important clinical observations. This is true of the umbilical arteries and of the normal and transplanted renal waveform, and so on.

The advantages of the RI in the determination of the renal transplant rejection have been reported.[27] In a series of papers, an RI of 0.7 was defined as normal renal impedance.[28] Acute hydronephrosis gives rise to an elevated RI, which has helped in the differentiation between caliectasis without obstruction and caliectasis caused by obstruction.

Systolic/Diastolic Ratio

Another index that has been applied to the study of the fetal circulation and umbilical and uterine arteries is the systolic/diastolic ratio (S/D). It is calculated simply by dividing the maximum systolic height of the Doppler waveform, f_{Dmax}, by the minimum diastolic height, f_{Dmin}, or

$$S/D = \frac{f_{Dmax}}{f_{Dmin}}. \qquad (21)$$

A major disadvantage of this index is when f_{Dmin} approaches ± 0, S/D tends to $\pm$ infinity and negative diastolic values cannot be expressed.

CLINICAL APPLICATIONS

The S/D has been widely used in obstetrics to quantitate the impedance of the placenta as reflected in the umbilical artery.[29] Absence or reversal of diastolic flow is a critical observation in the assessment of high-risk pregnancies.

The RI, PI, and S/D have been compared as applied to the umbilical artery waveform.[30] It was not possible to detect any difference between the different indices. Therefore it appears that the RI is the easiest to use and calculate and has no disadvantages compared with the alternatives.

Despite the voluminous literature on the value of PIs in the prediction of fetal compromise, a recent paper using meta–analysis of 15 studies of Doppler criteria showed positive predictive values of only 17 to 57 percent, which is similar to that reported for morphologic criteria alone.[31] Criteria using waveform analysis of the fetal internal carotid artery and aortic waveforms showed more promise in early studies. Thus, it has been concluded that no Doppler criterion has yet emerged as a clinically useful method to screen for IUGR.[31]

Laplace Transform

Another technique of feature extraction with specific application to the peripheral arterial system[32] is based on the description of the entire instantaneous peak velocity waveform, $v_{pk}(t) = cf_{Dpk}(t)/2\cos(\theta)f_o$. Unlike the crude pulsatility indices described before, this method allows for the reconstruction of the instantaneous peak velocity envelope. It does not, however, allow the reconstruction of the original velocity-time waveform.

The advantage of the Laplace transform method is that it models the properties of the arterial system (i.e., arterial stiffness, proximal lumen size, and distal impedance). The Fourier transform of the instantaneous peak velocity envelope over one cardiac cycle is computed first. The equivalent Laplace transform is then fitted in the least–squares sense to an arterial model of the form:

$$H(s) = \frac{1}{(s^2 + 2\delta\omega_o s + \omega_o^2)(s + \gamma)} \quad (22)$$

where $s = j\omega$ and the positions of the poles on the Argand diagram are determined by ω_o, γ, and δ. By equating the denominator of Equation 22 to zero, the three poles are found to be

$$\begin{aligned} s_1 &= -\gamma \\ s_{2,3} &= -\delta\omega_o \pm j\omega_o\sqrt{1 - \delta^2} \,. \end{aligned} \quad (23)$$

It has been postulated that γ, the real pole, is related to the degree of distal impedance.[32] Also, ω_o^2 is theoretically proportional to the elastic modulus of the wall of the arterial segment interrogated.[33] The position of the complex poles on the Argand diagram is dictated by δ and ω_o. The term δ, or the Laplace transform damping coefficient, was shown to be a function of the damping of the instantaneous peak velocity waveform caused by proximal stenosis.

CLINICAL APPLICATIONS

Preliminary observations[34] and a larger study[35] suggested that the Laplace transform damping is a sensitive indicator of iliac artery stenosis during the analysis of femoral artery Doppler signals. The PI was also computed in these studies and was found to indicate proximal disease but could not be used to grade the severity of iliac disease. In an extensive study,[36] the efficacy of the Laplace transform damping coefficient, δ, and PI, among other waveform shape indices, was assessed in detecting occlusive disease in peripheral arteries. The diagnostic accuracy of each index was determined from receiver operator characteristic curves. It was concluded that, in contrast to the earlier reports,[34,35] the Laplace transform did not prove to be superior to the other indices. Also, γ, the real pole, was shown to be uncorrelated with the amount of popliteal disease. In another paper,[37] it was concluded in a study of patients with multisegmental arterial disease that both PI and δ were equally good in the identification of aortoiliac disease, even when the superficial femoral artery was occluded. Because of the approximately equivalent diagnostic accuracy of these two indices, it seems that PI has the advantage of simplicity and ease of real-time calculation and would be the index of choice for the detection of arterial disease. None of the indices described thus far, however, is capable of accurately grading the severity of the lesion.

A variant of the Laplace transform technique just described has been used to detect IUGR by the analysis of flow in the descending thoracic aorta of the fetus.[38] The equivalent Laplace transform of the Fourier transform of the instantaneous peak velocity envelope was found in the form of a third-order polynomial:

$$H(s) = \frac{A + Bs}{1 + Cs + Ds^2 + Es^3} \qquad (24)$$

where $s = j\omega$. It was determined that C was the dominant coefficient, and this was used empirically to detect IUGR. A model was not developed to relate the changes in the coefficient, C, however, with any of the physiologic properties of the maternal–fetal arterial system.

DOPPLER STUDIES OF TUMOR FLOW AND THE ROLE OF COLOR-FLOW IMAGING

There have been multiple reports on the Doppler investigations of tumor flow characteristics. These include studies of liver tumors,[39] renal tumors,[40] breast tumors,[41–43] and ovarian tumors.[44,45] The recent addition of sensitive color flow has improved the detection of tumor vascularization considerably. These studies are either qualitative, such as the report of a basket appearance of vessels in hepatomas,[46] or quantitative, in which attempts have been made to estimate the Doppler shifts or velocities, or both, and to develop cut-off limits to differentiate benign from malignant tumors.[39,47] Although color flow may aid in the detection of hypervascularity and pattern recognition can be used to diagnose tumors, such qualitative uses for color flow vary between different machines, and new equipment improvements are increasing the signal-to-noise ratio. In the same way that formerly anechoic vessels show obvious color flow, tumors that appeared avascular on older equipment may now appear highly vascular. Because of this limitation, it would seem preferable to use color flow to recognize areas of abnormal vascularity and then to determine flow in them, using the velocity-time representation of the Doppler information. As is shown later, objective quantitative velocities can be used in clinical practice. The pathologic basis for the occurrence of these high-velocity Doppler shifts is considered to be arteriovenous shunting, a common finding in tumor vascularity.[48]

A further criterion that has been intensively investigated is the RI. This has been found to be lower in some tumors and is considered to be associated with the relative lack of muscle in the wall of tumor vessels. As can be seen in a series of studies from this institution,[39,40,47,48] however, the RI has failed to differentiate between benign and malignant tumors. This is in contrast to reports[44,45] that the RI can be used as a predictor of malignancy in ovarian tumors.

Liver Tumors

Focal liver masses are frequently found during sonography performed for benign reasons such as for the demonstration of gallstones. In addition, liver ultrasound is routinely requested in patients with known malignancies or in patients of high risk to develop hepatocellular carcinoma (HCC) because of cirrhosis or prior hepatitis B exposure, or both. The differential diagnosis of solid focal liver masses includes hemangiomas, focal fat, hepatomas, metastases, and several rare conditions such as hepatic cell adenoma and focal nodular hyperplasia. We have used color and duplex Doppler to help characterize liver tumors in 306 consecutive patients with focal liver lesions.[47] In 132 patients with pathologically proven diagnoses, there were 46 hepatic cell carcinomas and 86 metastases (Plate 10-1). Hemangiomas were more difficult to obtain with satisfactory confirmation, but 23 hemangiomas were considered to have been proved by ^{99m}Tc tagged red cell study, magnetic resonance imaging (MRI), or the computed tomography (CT) hemangioma protocol. In 43 other patients, there was no history of cancer, and the lesions were considered to be benign on the basis of stability during a minimum 2-year period. All patients were examined at a frequency of 3 MHz. The mean kilohertz shifts and standard deviations are shown in Table 10-1. The nonparametric Wilcoxon rank sum test revealed a statistically significant difference between HCC and metastases ($P < .001$) and between metastases and all benign lesions ($P < .001$).

Using a cut-off Doppler shift of 4.5 kHz, 32 hepatomas and four metastases provided a sensitivity of 70 percent and a specificity of 95 percent for distinguishing hepatomas

Table 10-1 Doppler Shifts in Liver Lesions

Types of Lesions	kHz ± SD
Hepatomas (HCC)	4.74 ± 1.74
Metastases	2.04 ± 1.68
Hemangiomas	0.53 ± 0.77
Other benign lesions	0.34 ± 0.77

from metastases. A lower cut-off of 2.5 kHz gave a 58 percent sensitivity but a 94 percent specificity for distinguishing malignant from benign lesions. The Pourcelot (resistive) indices were not significantly different.

Renal Masses

The vascularity of indeterminate renal masses in 70 patients was investigated prospectively with duplex ultrasound.[40] The peak systolic Doppler shift frequency obtained from the renal mass was used to attempt distinction between benign and malignant lesions. Using a criterion of a peak systolic Doppler shift frequency of 2.5 kHz or greater as evidence of neovascularity, 26 of 37 malignant lesions showed high Doppler shifts (70 percent sensitivity). Thirty-one of 33 lesions lacked high Doppler shifts (94 percent specificity). Both of the false-positive lesions were renal abscesses with obvious pyuria and peak frequencies of 3.0 and 3.7 kHz. The RIs were 0.70 for the tumors and 0.71 for the benign masses. These were not significantly different. We concluded that tumor vascularity in most malignant renal mass lesions gives rise to abnormal, high-frequency, Doppler-shifted signals that can aid the differential diagnosis of renal masses.

Breast Masses

Several previous authors have reported the presence of neovascularity in breast cancer.[42,43] In another series, more than 300 palpable breast masses have been examined using CW Doppler at 10 MHz.[41] Surgical and pathologic proof was available in 200 breast masses, of which 113 were benign and 87 malignant. An abnormal examination consisted of asymmetry exceeding 2 kHz between the mass and its mirror image in the other breast. This criterion provided a sensitivity of 78 percent and a specificity of 71 percent for the differentiation of benign from malignant masses. Compared with the results of previous authors who reported much higher sensitivities and specificities,[42] these figures do not provide adequate utility for Doppler as a diagnostic modality. Therefore it was decided[41] to investigate whether the presence of Doppler signals was predictive of a worse prognosis. An abnormal Doppler result was correlated with known predictors of prognosis. To increase the number of breast cancers, study results from Bristol, England, were also analyzed.[42]

Doppler signals were abnormal in 68 of 87 breast cancers (78 percent) and normal in 19 breast cancers. Abnormal Doppler signals were present in 96.3 percent of patients with positive lymph nodes, 93.3 percent of patients with tumors greater than 2.5 cm, 100 percent (15 of 15) of patients with residual disease after surgery, 97 percent of patients with advanced disease at presentation, and 100 percent (17 of 17) of patients with tumor recurrence. It was concluded that tumor-dependent neovascularity (as detected by continuous-wave Doppler) is predictive of more aggressive breast cancers.[41]

Ovarian Tumors

A review of patients at Yale presenting with palpable pelvic masses was performed to develop criteria to help characterize malignant from benign adnexal masses using endovaginal color-flow imaging (Taylor, unpublished data). To date, 95 women with palpable pelvic masses have been examined. Ovarian volume has been estimated, and morphologic features including septations and mural nodules have been evaluated. Pulse Doppler interrogation was also performed (Plate 10-2). Pathology has become available in 27 patients. Twenty were benign and seven were malignant, of which three were stage I ovarian carcinoma. Using size as a criterion of ovarian abnormality, 18 ml was regarded as the upper limit of normal for a premenopausal patient and 8 ml for postmenopausal ovary. Sixteen of 20 (80 percent of benign tumors) had an ovarian vol-

ume outside the normal range (mean volume, 74 ml). All seven carcinomas (100 percent) had a volume outside the normal range (mean volume, 603 ml). All seven carcinomas and 13 of the benign lesions (65 percent) showed irregular solid components or septations, or both. Doppler criteria showed peak systolic velocities of greater than 25 cm/s in six of seven carcinomas (sensitivity, 86 percent) but only in four benign masses (specificity, 80 percent). An RI of less than 0.5 was not a sensitive predictor of malignancy because it occurred in only three of seven carcinomas (sensitivity, 43 percent) and also in two benign lesions (specificity, 90 percent). Even this overestimated the specificity of a low RI. The RI for a normal corpus luteum is 0.44 ± 0.09. Luteal flow frequently was persistent into the early days of the next cycle, but repeat scans were performed to document normal cycling. This allowed recognition of luteal flow so that these patients did not go to surgery. In this preliminary work, it was concluded that a peak systolic velocity greater than 25 cm/s in an enlarged complex adnexal mass was the best predictor of malignancy. A low RI was not a sensitive indicator of ovarian cancer.

CONCLUSIONS

In the past decade, there have been dramatic improvements in ultrasound image quality. It seems unlikely that further improvements of the same magnitude can be made in the future without extrinsic methods of increasing the signal-to-noise ratio, such as with the use of contrast agents. Compared with these improvements in image quality, quantitative analysis of Doppler data has shown slow progress. It seems probable that this will be the area in which considerable effort will be expended to obtain quantitative information that will greatly increase the clinical value of Doppler-derived parameters.

REFERENCES

1. Gill RW: Measurement of blood flow by ultrasound: accuracy and sources of error. Ultrasound Med Biol 11:625, 1985
2. Wilson LS, Dadd MJ, Gill RW: Automatic vessel tracking and measurement for Doppler studies. Ultrasound Med Biol 16:645, 1990
3. Evans DH: On the measurement of the mean velocity of blood flow over the cardiac cycle using Doppler ultrasound. Ultrasound Med Biol 11:735, 1985
4. Cobbold RSC, Veltink PH, Johnson KW: Influence of beam profile and degree of insonation on the CW Doppler ultrasound spectrum and mean velocity. IEEE Trans Sonics Ultrason 30:364, 1983
5. Newhouse VL, Eherenwald AR, Johnson GF: The effect of Rayleigh scattering and frequency-dependent absorption on the output spectrum of Doppler blood flowmeters. p. 1181. In White D, Brown RE (eds): Ultrasound in Medicine 3B. Plenum Press, New York, 1977
6. Holland SK, Orphanoudakis SC, Jaffe CC: Frequency-dependent attenuation effects in pulsed Doppler ultrasound: experimental results. IEEE Trans Biomed Eng 31:626, 1984
7. Gill RW: Performance of the mean frequency Doppler modulator. Ultrasound Med Biol 5: 237, 1979
8. Green PS: Spectral broadening of acoustic reverberation in Doppler-shift fluid flowmeters. J Acoust Soc Am 36:1383, 1964
9. Gerzberg L, Meindl JD: Mean frequency estimator with applications in ultrasonic Doppler flowmeters. p. 1173. In White D, Brown RE (eds): Ultrasound in Medicine 3B. Plenum Press, New York, 1977
10. Newhouse VL, Varner LW, Bendick PJ: Geometrical spectrum broadening in ultrasonic Doppler systems. IEEE Trans Biomed Eng 24:478, 1977
11. Newhouse VL, Furgason ES, Johnson GF, Wolf DA: The dependence of ultrasound Doppler bandwidth on beam geometry. IEEE Trans Sonics Ultrason 27:50, 1980
12. Eik-Nes SH, Marsal K, Kristoffersen K: Methodology and basic problems related to blood flow studies in the human fetus. Ultrasound Med Biol 8:605, 1984
13. Gill RW, Kossoff G, Warren PS, Garrett WJ: Umbilical venous flow in normal and complicated pregnancy. Ultrasound Med Biol 10: 349, 1984
14. Moriyasu F, Ban N, Nishida O et al: Clinical application of an ultrasonic duplex system in the quantitative measurement of portal blood flow. J Clin Ultrasound 14:579, 1986
15. Evans DH, McDicken WN, Skidmore R, Woodcock JP: Doppler Ultrasound: Physics, Instrumentation, and Clinical Applications. Wiley, New York, 1989
16. Evans DH: On the measurement of the mean velocity of blood flow over the cardiac cycle using Doppler ultrasound. Ultrasound Med Biol 11:735, 1985
17. Sabbá C, Weltin G, Cicchetti DV et al: Observer variability in echo-Doppler measurements of portal flow in cirrhotic patients and normal volunteers. Gastroenterology 98: 1603, 1990
18. Sabbá C, Ferraioli G, Genecin P et al: Evaluation of post-prandial hyperemia in superior mesenteric artery and portal vein in healthy and cirrhotic humans: an operator-blind echo Doppler study. Hepatology 13:714, 1991
19. Hottinger CF, Meindl JD: Blood flow measurement using the attenuation-compensated volume flowmeter. Ultrason Imaging 1:1, 1979
20. Fu C-C, Gerzberg L: Annular arrays for quantitative pulsed Doppler ultrasonic flowmeters. Ultrason Imaging 5:1, 1983
21. Nichols WW, O'Rourke MF (eds): MacDonald's Blood Flow in Arteries: Theoretical, Experimental and Clinical Principles. Lea & Febinger, Philadelphia, 1990
22. Gosling RG, Dunbar G, King DH et al: The quantitative analysis of occlusive peripheral arterial disease by a non-intrusive ultrasonic technique. Angiology 22:52, 1971
23. Gosling RG, King DH: Arterial assessment by Doppler-shift ultrasound. Proc Soc Med 67:447, 1974
24. Rigsby C, Taylor KJW, Welton G et al: Renal allografts in acute rejection: evaluation using duplex sonography. Radiology 158:375, 1986
25. Taylor KJW, Marks WH: Use of Doppler imaging for evaluation of dysfunction in renal allografts. AJR 155:536, 1990
26. Pourcelot L: Applications cliniques de l'exa-

men Doppler transcutane. p. 780. In Peronneau P (ed): Velocimetrie Ultrasonore Doppler. INSERM 34, Paris, 1974

27. Rifkin MD, Needleman L, Pasto ME et al: Evaluation of renal transplant rejection by duplex Doppler examination: value of the resistive index. AJR 148:759, 1987

28. Platt JF, Rubin JM, Ellis JH, DiPietro MA: Duplex Doppler ultrasound of the kidney: differentiation of obstructive from nonobstructive dilation. Radiology 171:515, 1989

29. Fitzgerald DE, Stuart B, Drumm JE et al: The assessment of the feto-placental circulation with continuous wave Doppler ultrasound. Ultrasound Med Biol 10:371, 1984

30. Thompson RS, Trudinger BJ, Cooke CM: A comparison of Doppler ultrasound waveform indices in the umbilical artery—1. Indices derived from the maximum velocity waveform. Ultrasound Med Biol 12:835, 1986

31. Benson CB, Doubilet PM: Doppler criteria for intrauterine growth retardation: predictive values. J Ultrasound Med 7:655, 1988

32. Skidmore R, Woodcock JP: Physiological interpretation of Doppler-shift waveforms—I. Theoretical considerations. Ultrasound Med Biol 6:7, 1980

33. Skidmore R, Woodcock JP: Physiological interpretation of Doppler-shift waveforms—II. Validation of the Laplace transform method for characterization of the common femoral blood-velocity/time waveform. Ultrasound Med Biol 6:219, 1980

34. Skidmore R, Woodcock JP, Wells PNT et al: Physiological interpretation of Doppler-shift waveforms—III. Clinical results. Ultrasound Med Biol 6:227, 1980

35. Baird RN, Bird DR, Clifford PC et al: Upstream stenosis. Arch Surg 115:1316, 1980

36. Johnston KW, Kassam M, Koers J et al: Comparative study of four methods for quantifying Doppler ultrasound waveforms from the femoral artery. Ultrasound Med Biol 10: 1, 1984

37. Junger M, Chapman BLW, Underwood CJ, Charlesworth D: A comparison between two types of waveform analysis in patients with multisegmental arterial disease. Br J Surg 71: 345, 1984

38. Stone PR, Skidmore R, Baker JD, Stirrat GM: Fetal Doppler shift waveforms in intrauterine growth retardation: Laplace transform analysis technique. Ultrasound Med Biol 16:773, 1990

39. Taylor KJW, Ramos I, Morse S et al: Focal liver masses: differential diagnosis with pulsed Doppler US. Radiology 164:643, 1987

40. Kier R, Taylor KJW, Feyock AL, Ramos IM: Renal masses: characterization with Doppler US. Radiology 176:703, 1990

41. Scoutt L, Ramos IM, Taylor KJW et al: CW Doppler examinations of breast masses. Radiology 169:21, 1988

42. Burns PN, Halliwell M, Webb AJ et al: Ultrasonic Doppler studies of the breast. Ultrasound Med Biol 8:127, 1982

43. Minasian H, Bamber JC: A preliminary assessment of an ultrasonic Doppler method of the study of blood flow in human breast cancer. Ultrasound Med Biol 8:357, 1982

44. Bourne T, Campbell S, Steer C et al: Transvaginal color flow imaging: a possible new screening technique for ovarian cancer. Br Med J 229:1367, 1989

45. Kurjak A, Zalud I, Alfirevic Z, Jurkovic D: The assessment of abnormal pelvic blood flow by transvaginal color and pulsed Doppler. Ultrasound Med Biol 16:437, 1990

46. Tanaka S, Kitamura T, Fujita M et al: Color Doppler flow imaging of liver tumors. AJR 154:509, 1990

47. Hammers LW, Case CL, Reinhold CY et al: Pulsed Doppler US of focal liver masses. Radiology 181:225, 1991

48. Taylor KJW, Ramos I, Carter D et al: Correlation of Doppler US tumor signals with neovascular morphologic features. Radiology 166:57, 1988

11

Ultrasound Picture Archiving and Communication Systems

H. K. Huang

A picture archiving and communication system (PACS) has many definitions depending on the user's perspective. It can be as simple as a film digitizer connected to a display station managing a small database, or it can be as complex as a total hospital image management system. Generally speaking, a PACS consists of acquisition, storage, and display subsystems integrated by various digital networks and a database management system.

PACS INFRASTRUCTURE

The PACS infrastructure[1] consists of a basic skeleton of hardware components including image acquisition interfaces, storage devices, host computers, communication networks, and display systems. These components are integrated by standardized, flexible software subsystems. The important software subsystems include communication, database and storage management, job scheduling, interprocessor communication, error handling, and network monitoring. The software modules of the infrastructure have sufficient understanding and cooperation at a system level such that the components work together as a team rather than as individual computers connected in a network. The ultrasound PACS infrastructure design can be physically compartmentalized into five classes of computer/processor units connected by different network circuits: (1) ultrasound acquisition devices, (2) acquisition computers, (3) cluster controllers, (4) database servers, and (5) display workstations. Figure 11-1 shows the interrelationship between these units.

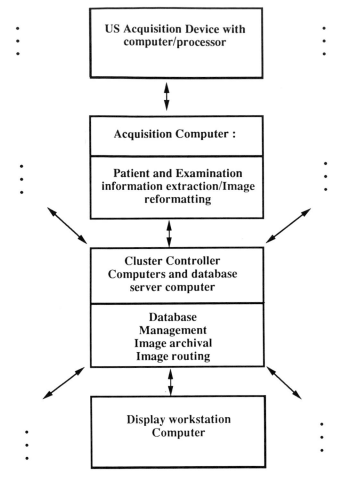

Fig. 11-1 Ultrasound PACS infrastructure design with five classes of computers connected by different network circuits.

Acquisition Computer

Let us assume that an ultrasound image has been acquired and digitized from the ultrasound device. An acquisition computer is used as an intermediate buffer for this digitized image between the ultrasound device and the cluster controller. An acquisition computer has many functions including (1) accepting images from the ultrasound acquisition device and serving as a buffer; (2) reformatting an image to a standard format (e.g., the ACR/NEMA [American College of Radiology/National Electrical Manufac-

turers Association] standard)[2]; (3) acquiring patient demographic and examination-related information; (4) compiling image and text information into a data file; and (5) transmitting the data file to the cluster controller for long-term archival and for routing to the display station. For ultrasound application, the acquisition computer can be a low-cost IBM-compatible PC.

The method for sending images from an ultrasound device to an acquisition computer is a peer-to-peer communication. In operation, image transfers can be initiated either by the ultrasound device (a push operation) or by the acquisition computer (a pull operation). Generally speaking, the pull mode is the preferred mode of operation because the acquisition computer can be programmed to reschedule image transfers if a failure occurs to the computer or to the ultrasound device. However, almost all ultrasound devices do not have sufficient data buffering on the imaging system for the pull operation to function properly and efficiently. Therefore, the push mode by the ultrasound device is the one commonly used.

Cluster Controller and Database Server

Data files from the acquisition computer are sent to a cluster controller. A cluster controller is logically defined as a group of computers with software to perform various functions pertinent to image acquisition, image routing, archiving management, and system monitoring and reliability. An ultrasound cluster (or a pediatric radiology or a chest radiology cluster) could exist as a logical entity within the PACS infrastructure.

A cluster controller is comprised of a host computer, a mass storage device for long-term archival (e.g., an optical disk library), and a fast magnetic disk for short-term storage. One major function of the cluster controller is automatically to combine images from the current ultrasound examination with historic images and forward them to a display workstation for review. Certain intelligence needs to be incorporated into the cluster controller database server software to perform this task.

Display Station

The display station is the component by which physicians interact with the PACS. A station includes communication, database, display, resource management, and processing software. The fundamental operations

are case preparation, case selection, image arrangement, interpretation, documentation, and case presentations. In the case of an ultrasound station, medium resolution 1k × 1k monitors with the capability of split screen and ciné mode are sufficient for most of the clinical applications.

System Networking

Three types of digital networks can be used for ultrasound image transmission between components in the PACS infrastructure[3]: the low-speed Ethernet (10 megabytes/s signaling rate); the medium-speed (100 megabytes/s) fiber distributed data interface (FDDI); and the high-speed (1 gigabyte/s) proprietary network circuits. The most commonly used communication protocol is the transmission control protocol/internet protocol (TCP/IP). Process coordination between tasks running on different computers in the infrastructure is essential in system networking. This coordination of process running either on the same computer or on different computers is accomplished by using interprocessor communication methods implemented with socket level software interfacing to the TCP/IP.

Some Important PACS Design Concepts

STANDARDIZATION

Use of industrial hardware and software standard for PACS development has two advantages: minimizing the development of software, and increasing the portability of the system to other computer platforms. Some current industrial standards are (1) UNIX computer operating system, (2) TCP/IP communication protocol, (3) structured query database language (SQL), (4) ACR-NEMA standard for radiologic image communication, (5) C programming language, (6) X-windows user interface, and (7) ASCII text representation for message passing.

OPEN ARCHITECTURE

Open architecture is a necessary condition for communication between components in the PACS infrastructure. An open network design architecture allows the use of standards for message, data, and image exchange between heterogeneous systems. PACS infrastructure consists of many heterogeneous systems; an open architecture design using industrial standards yields a higher probability of success for PACS implementation.

ULTRASOUND IMAGE ACQUISITION

Image Data

To implement an ultrasound PACS, the first step is to acquire digital images from the ultrasound scanner. There are two methods for acquiring digital ultrasound images: directly in digital format or through the video board. In the direct digital method, the digital ultrasound image is acquired before it is written onto the video circuit. This method is preferable because it preserves the image quality in the sense that the digital image does not have to be converted to video signals and then back to digital signal. However, currently, most manufacturers do not support this digital interface.

The second method is to digitize the analog signal from the video board in the ultrasound device. This method can be easily accomplished with a frame-grabber. A typical scenario is as follows (Fig. 11-2). A microcomputer (e.g., a PC with a frame-grabber and some on-board image memory) can be used as the acquisition computer. Within the ultrasound device, the digital image is stored as a $512 \times 512 \times 8$-bit image, which is converted continuously into a display video image. The video signal is routed to both the ultrasound device display monitor and the multiformat camera or a videotape recorder. The video signal can be interrupted from one of the three video sources and digitized by the A/D converter in the frame-grabber. The digitized image is routed to the on-board image memory for temporary storage.

It is important that the digital image acquisition process should be as automatic as possible. One method to accomplish this is to use the film printer exposure signal as a PC interrupt signal for capturing the image from the video line. This signal interrupts the running program in the microcomputer and, in $\frac{1}{30}$ second, places the digital image currently on the ultrasound display into the on-board image memory. Meanwhile, the PC prepares the frame-grabber for the next image. Theoretically, if the image memory is large enough, the PC can continuously digitize ultrasound images without any interruption.

Once the image acquisition is completed, all images can be transferred to the cluster controller computer through the Ethernet TCP/IP communication protocol. Figure 11-2 shows the components in the ultrasound acquisition computer and their connections to the ultrasound device and the cluster controller computer.

Patient and Examination Information

Patient and examination information related to the images can be extracted by either of two methods. The first method is to use a serial interface in the acquisition computer connecting to the ultrasound device. When the patient and examination data are entered by the operator to the ultrasound device during examination, these data can also be sent automatically to the acquisition computer through the interface. Communication software in the ultrasound device and in the acquisition computer have to be written to establish the hand-shaking between these two units. To use this method of interface, cooperation from the ultrasound manufacturer is necessary.

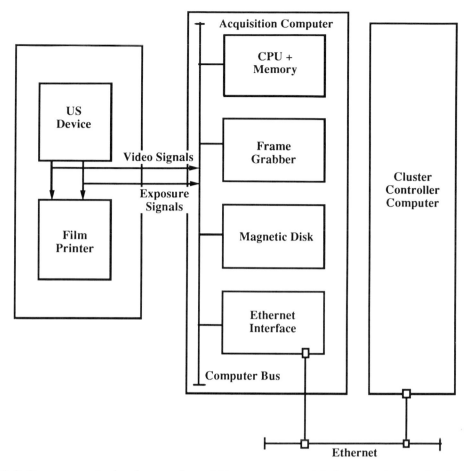

Fig. 11-2 Components in the ultrasound acquisition computer and their connections to the ultrasound device and the cluster controller computer.

The second method is to extract the information directly from the digital ultrasound image captured in the frame-grabber image memory. In ultrasound images, patient and examination information appear on identical relative locations in every image and are represented by a limited character set of a certain font (e.g., a 5 × 7 pixel matrix). We can use a standard character recognition algorithm to identify these characters and to compile and append them with the images to form a complete data file. The disadvantages of this method are that the locations of the characters and the character sets may be different in different ultrasound units.

INTERFACE ULTRASOUND ACQUISITION TO PACS: AN EXAMPLE

Ultrasound Image and Text Acquisition

The Department of Radiological Sciences at UCLA implemented a pediatric radiology PACS acquisition, storage, and display system in 1987.[4] The acquisition included a computed radiographic (CR) system (PCR-901, Philips Medical Systems, USA), a laser film digitizer (Konica, Japan), and a magnetic resonance (MR) system (FONAR B3000, USA). In the beginning, a direct ultrasound interface to the PACS was not established. Ultrasound images were digitized from ultrasound films with the laser scanner. This method of integration of ultrasound images into PACS was neither sufficient nor efficient. There were three ultrasound units in the pediatric radiology section, and it was time-consuming for the technologist to digitize every ultrasound film with the laser film scanner, especially because nine images usually were printed onto a single film. A direct interface was necessary to collect images and patient data automatically, with minimum human interaction.[5]

Compared with the existing CR and MR acquisition systems, ultrasound devices posed new problems in acquisition and PACS integration. Ultrasound devices are (1) portable, (2) more numerous than CR or MR, (3) not based on dedicated minicomputer systems, and (4) usually without any digital image storage unit such as a magnetic disk. The life of ultrasound images within the ultrasound device is short—they are available only until the operator pushes the print button for exposing film (Fig. 11-2). During an ultrasound examination, many images (about 20 to 30) come in a relatively short time interval (about 15 to 30 minutes). During this time, the ultrasonographer is totally absorbed in patient examination and cannot be interrupted easily. Therefore, the image capturing time has to be coincident with the time when the print button is pushed. Based on these differences in operational conditions, we decided to digitize the analog signal directly from the video board in the ultrasound device.[6]

An IBM-PC/XT with a magnetic disk was configured with a video frame-grabber board (MATROX) with four 512 × 512 × 8-bit memories and a network interface board (Excelan Ethernet board). The ultrasound film printer exposure signal was used as a PC interrupt signal for capturing the image from the video line. This signal interrupted the

running program in the PC and, in $\frac{1}{30}$ second, placed the image currently on the ultrasound display onto one of four frame-grabber memories. Images could be transferred to the magnetic disk afterward. The PC prepared the frame memory to act as a four-element circular queue. For patient information extraction, we used the character recognition algorithm to identify characters on the image. After this character set was extracted from each image, it was used to identify the image. This information was appended as a portion of the examination header record. Collection of all images and the header record formed the complete patient ultrasound image file.

Image Transfer Between the Capture Computer and the Network Computer

The image file was transferred to the PACS network computer one image at a time using the file transfer protocol (FTP) utility based on the Ethernet TCP/IP. Because the PC was a single-task machine and we used the FTP facility, we could not interrupt the process during image transfer. If, during the image transfer, another ultrasound image on the display monitor was ready to be digitized and the frame-grabber failed to serve its function immediately, we might lose this image. This is because new ultrasound images might overwrite the image on the display monitor. To minimize the potential for image loss during transfer, we adopted a polling strategy between the PC and the PACS network computer as follows. After successfully transferring one image to the PACS network computer, the PC polled the ultrasound device exposure latch to see if a new image had been generated in the display monitor during the image transmission. If present, the PC initiated the digitization, sent the digitized image to the magnetic disk as a temporary buffer, and polled the exposure latch again. If there was no new activity in the exposure latch for more than 3 minutes, image transfer between the PC and the network computer resumed. After transferring the complete image file to the network computer, the PC deleted the image file from the magnetic disk to save storage space for the next image files. The PC also recalled and served those new images temporarily stored in the disk to form new complete patient image files. Although this polling scheme could minimize the loss of images, it required the cooperation of the ultrasound operator. If too many new images were acquired in a short time, the power of the PC might not be able to keep up with the demands of both image transfer and the forming of complete image files. In this situation, the ultrasound operator had to control the new image flow to the ultrasound video monitor manually. This method of interfacing ultrasound image acquisition to PACS networks was completed in 1989.[6]

ULTRASOUND PACS DESIGN

The design of a large-scale ultrasound PACS at UCLA[7] will append two main components, image acquisition and image display, in the existing UCLA PACS infrastructure.

Specifications

At UCLA, ultrasound examinations at the Department of Radiological Sciences are performed mainly at two locations: the Center for Health Sciences (CHS) for in-patient services, and Medical Plaza (MP) for out-patient services. The distance between the two locations is about 1 km, and they are connected by fiber optic and Ethernet cables. Images from other examinations such as computed tomography (CT), MR, and CR are routinely transferred through either Ethernet, FDDI, or Ultranet communication circuits using the TCP/IP protocol.

Table 11-1 shows the total number of ultrasound devices in both locations and the estimation of numbers of examinations and images generated. In this estimation, we assume one patient study consists of about 650 images, each with a size of 512 × 512 × 8 bits. Twelve ultrasound devices generate approximately 46 examinations, 2,300 images, and 575 megabytes per day. As a comparison, a CT scanner generates about 15 examinations and 300 megabytes per day.

The overall architecture of the ultrasound PACS module connected to the existing infrastructure is shown in Figure 11-3. Ultra-

Table 11-1 Number of Ultrasound Devices and Estimation of Examinations and Images Generated per Day

	No. of Ultrasound Devices	Exams/Day	Images/Day	Storage MB/Day
Center for Health Sciences (in-patient)				
Ultrasound section	5	15	750	187.5
Mobile	1	2	100	25.0
Total	6	17	850	212.5
Medical Plaza				
Ultrasound section	3	12	600	150.0
Mental Health	2	15	750	187.5
Endoscopy	1	2	100	25.0
Total	6	29	1,450	362.5
Grand Total	12	46	2,300	575.0

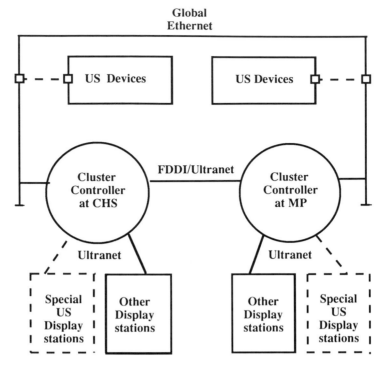

Fig. 11-3 Overall architecture of the ultrasound PACS module connected to the infrastructure. (——), in existence; (----) planning.

sound images will be acquired from ultrasound devices and transferred to the two existing cluster controllers at CHS and MP through a global Ethernet using the TCP/IP protocol. At the cluster controller computers, ultrasound images will be grouped according to body regions and appended to the patient image files, which also contain images from other examinations. The patient image files will then be transmitted to existing display stations. At the same time, self-contained ultrasound image files will also be sent to specially designed ultrasound display stations for interpretation. The exchange of ultrasound images between the out-patient facility at the MP and the in-patient facility at the CHS will be taken care of automatically by the cluster controller's database management system, based on the patient status.

Image Acquisition and Interface Component

The interface of ultrasound devices to the PACS infrastructure can be accomplished through a specially designed interface device provided by the manufacturer (Advanced Technology Laboratories, USA). The interface component consists of a three-way foot switch, a local magnetic disk, an Ethernet circuit, and a microprocessor connected to the ultrasound device. Figure 11-4 shows a prototype unit being tested in our department. In operation, switch 1 initiates the digitization and stores the image in the frame buffer. Switch 2 protects the image in the buffer from overwriting. Switch 3 transmits the image to a local disk for temporary storage. When the ultrasound device is not scanning, the cluster controller initiates a com-

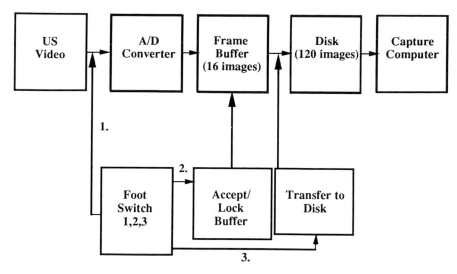

Fig. 11-4 Method of acquiring digital images from ultrasound video signals through a foot pedal with three switches.

mand to transfer the ultrasound image from the local disk to the cluster controller's disk.

Ultrasound Display Station

Ultrasound images can be displayed by two methods. First, they can be appended to the complete patient image file at the cluster controller, which also contains images from other examinations. A physician can review images from any examinations including ultrasound through a 1k or 2k display station already in clinical operation. Alternatively, ultrasound images can be grouped as a special procedure examination and displayed at a specially designed ultrasound display station. The ultrasound display station is different from other display stations in that the former requires pseudocolor to display flow images. Also, ciné mode is needed for displaying dynamic studies. These two features are important in the design of the special ultrasound display station that is being developed in our department. We are currently in the final stage of completing the ultrasound PACS design.

SUMMARY

In this chapter, we discussed the concept of PACS infrastructure and the methods of implementing an ultrasound PACS. An ultrasound PACS differs from other radiologic PACS modules in several aspects. First, ultrasound image acquisition requires the interaction from the operator to initiate the image capture process. Second, ultrasound display requires pseudocolor to show flow images. Third, ultrasound examinations include dynamic studies that generate many images in real-time. The last feature is difficult to achieve even with current technology. One method is to explore video transmission, storage, and display technology. We have researched and implemented a fiber optic broadband video system for transmitting, archiving, and displaying CT and MR images in real-time. This system connects three CT and three MR scanners in three buildings including the CHS and the MP over a distance of about 2.5 km.[8] We believe this technology can be extended for real-time video ultrasound image transmission, archiving, and display.

ACKNOWLEDGMENTS

This research was partially supported by Public Health Service grant P01 CA 51198 from the USA National Cancer Institute, Department of Health and Human Services.

REFERENCES

1. Huang HK, Taira RK: PACS infrastructure design. AJR 158:743, 1992
2. ACR-NEMA Digital Imaging and Communication Standard. Publication 300. National Electrical Manufacturers Association, Washington, DC, 1985
3. Huang HK, Lou SL, Cho SL et al: Radiologic image communication methods. AJR 155:183, 1990
4. Taira RK, Mankovich NJ, Boechat MI et al: Design and implementation of a picture archiving and communication system (PACS) for pediatric radiology. AJR 150:1117, 1988
5. Lou SL, Huang HK, Mankovich NJ et al: A CT/MR/US picture archiving and communication system. p. 31. In Schneider RH (ed): SPIE Medical Imaging III, Bellingham, Washington, 1989
6. Park KS, Madachy RJ, Taira RK: Implementation of automatic digital ultrasonic image acquisition on a microcomputer. p. 83. In Schneider RH (ed): SPIE Medical Imaging III, Bellingham, Washington, 1989
7. Weinberg WS, Tessler FN, Gant EG et al: Development and implementation of ultrasonic picture archiving and communication system. p. 37. In Schneider RH (ed): SPIE Medical Imaging IV, Bellingham, Washington, 1990
8. Huang HK, Tecotsky RH, Bazzill T: A fiberoptic broadband CT/MR video communication system. J Digital Imaging 5:20, 1992

12

Impact of Safety Considerations on Ultrasound Equipment Design and Use

Marvin C. Ziskin
Thomas L. Szabo

Although much work remains to be done to measure and understand potential bioeffects induced by ultrasound, it is clear that the two dominant mechanisms are heating and transient cavitation. These mechanisms are known to occur at high intensity levels. In fact, high-intensity ultrasound is used deliberately to produce these effects for beneficial results. In the 0.8- to 3-MHz range, localized heating caused by ultrasound is used to promote healing. In hyperthermia applications, high intensities of ultrasound are applied to the skin surface or to soft tissue sites in the body for the selective destruction (through heat) of malignant tissue. Lithotripters use high-amplitude pressure waves to break up stones in vivo.

GENERAL APPROACH

Ultrasound-Induced Bioeffects

At the lower levels of power and relatively higher frequencies used in diagnostic applications, no deleterious effects have ever been reported. However, subtle or long-term delayed effects would not be obvious and might go undetected. So although ultrasound has been used diagnostically for many millions of examinations without any known adverse effects, the possibility for induced bioeffects is not ruled out. A reasonable approach to dealing with these uncertainties is to concentrate on controlling the two identified main bioeffect mechanisms and to continue further refinements in computations of bioeffects modeling and in vivo data gathering. In particular, the question of where and how to draw the line between diagnostic and therapeutic ultrasound levels needs to be addressed. Overviews and details of ultrasound bioeffects can be found by reference to other publications.[1-3]

Thermal effects are directly related to the absorption of the tissues in the region being insonified. Ideally, given the characteristics of the insonifying beam and the acoustic properties and locations of the overlying and target tissue, the local temperature rise can be predicted. Practically, however, the many possible imaging views and the variations among people being imaged—their body types and differences in tissue perfusion—make accurate individualistic prediction difficult. Exposure time is also important when the incoming energy is greater than the capability of perfused tissue to dissipate it; in this case, temperature rise increases with the length of exposure time to some thermal limit. Fortunately, there is no evidence that any of the effects of ultrasound are cumulative from examination to examination as is true for ionizing radiation.

Transient cavitation effects have been well characterized for unbounded nucleated water. Unlike heating, cavitation obeys a threshold law for bubbles present in unbounded water. Given the right match between bubble size and insonifying frequency, transient cavitation has been shown in water at both lithotripsy and diagnostic intensities. Whether the body and its tissues provide appropriate conditions for cavitation to occur is still under investigation. Several complicating factors are whether nucleation (bubble) sites of the appropriate size exist in the body and how tissue viscosity, structure, and boundaries affect the conditions for cavitation. Cavitation events are highly localized and difficult to detect in vivo. The cavitation threshold for bubbles in water is

approximately[4] the peak rarefractional pressure (MPa) divided by the square root of center frequency (MHz). Unlike lithotripsy applications, which combine high amplitudes and low frequencies, diagnostic applications have higher frequencies and lower amplitudes, which lead to higher thresholds. Furthermore, the presence of intervening tissue in the acoustic path diminishes the pressure amplitude in most diagnostic applications.

Risk Versus Benefit

Ideally the clinician should have a direct and meaningful indication of the likelihood of an adverse effect on a sensitive anatomic site within the individual being imaged for the particular ultrasound mode being used. Although complete accuracy is not now possible, a reasonable worst case estimate has been proposed[2,5] to give clinicians a conservative estimate of the likelihood of both thermally and cavitationally mediated effects so that appropriate action can be taken. These real-time predictions can be helpful to a clinician making a risk/benefit decision, as described in more detail later in this chapter. Most likely, this decision will be based mainly on the patient's condition and the relative safety of using ultrasound compared with other diagnostic modalities.

The "As Low As Reasonably Achievable" Principle

The "as low as reasonably achievable" principle (ALARA)[2,5] approach to ultrasound output control makes good common sense. It is considered prudent in medical practice that if there is any doubt as to what to do, do whatever is least dangerous to the patient. "Achievable" in this context is obtaining the necessary quality diagnostic information. If the sought-after information is not obtained because of an assumed improvement in safety, the consequences may be more hazardous for the patient; this factor needs to be considered in making the risk/benefit decision. In many cases, the diagnostic equipment being used may not be capable of producing a significant bioeffect. These arguments point to the necessity of providing the user with more real-time information about the capability of the imaging system to operate at levels known to cause identified bioeffects and with general guidelines about risk/benefit decisions and clinical use of the equipment.

Clinicians using present commercially available diagnostic ultrasound equipment are usually not aware of the acoustic output levels used. Even though they normally use good judgment and apply the ALARA principle, clinicians have no idea, in an absolute sense, whether their operation of the equipment is capable of producing a potentially "risky" situation. In cases where there is no possibility of harm, minimizing acoustic output would not have any significance for biologic effects. Thus, the clinician applies the ALARA principle as a conservative measure for patient safety without knowing the necessity or effectiveness of his or her actions.

INSTRUMENT ACOUSTIC OUTPUT INFORMATION

Complicating Factors

Determination of the potential risk of using diagnostic ultrasound equipment is difficult because of the growing complexity of the instruments available and the many ways the instruments can be applied. Some of the ultrasound scanners have more than 100,000 possible modes that are user-selectable[6]; this is a consequence of different combinations of front panel control settings affecting acoustic output. Not only are these systems used for different clinical applications, but for each application, there are several different imaging views and windows. Furthermore, the patients being imaged vary greatly in individual characteristics, body type, age, degree of health, and so on. Finally, acoustic output measurements are made by manufacturers under ideal water tank conditions, and the acoustic output levels existing at particular insonified locations in an individual are never known accurately.

Bioeffect Endpoint-Directed Approaches

Because of the difficulties just discussed, and the growing realization that acoustic output data presently supplied by manufacturers are not adequately helpful in making real-time risk/benefit decisions in clinical situations, simplified approaches based on bioeffect endpoints have emerged. One approach currently being considered by the International Electrotechnical Commission is based on the safety classification of ultrasound fields. According to this scheme, all ultrasound equipment would be categorized in two or more classes based on the capability of the equipment to generate a temperature rise or cavitation index exceeding defined threshold levels. Although the conditions under which these thresholds are to be determined have not been worked out, there is an implied worst-case assessment. A consensus is growing[2,5] that there may be a "safe" class of ultrasound imaging devices whose output falls below minimum thresholds for temperature rise.

For equipment capable of exceeding the minimum thresholds, questions remain as to what are the appropriate actions to take in specific circumstances. There is now no provision in this scheme for equipment rated in higher threshold classes to determine the conditions and applications for which the thresholds are exceeded or the resulting consequences.

Another approach to the risk/benefit dilemma has been proposed[5] for equipment or modes exceeding minimum thermal and mechanical (cavitation) indices; a real-time display of these indices is required. The thermal index is the ratio of the time-averaged power (or other power parameter) divided by the power necessary to raise the target tissue temperature by 1°C, based on thermal models. The mechanical (cavitation) index is based on a derated rarefractional pressure (MPa) divided by the square root of center frequency (MHz).

The display of indices would provide the user with real-time feedback in a more direct and understandable manner to aid in the application of the ALARA principle. An important component of the output display method is education of users of the equipment on the limitations of and guidelines for the use of indices and the appropriate considerations needed for risk/benefit decisions when the minimum thresholds are exceeded. These indices are estimates for different applications, and they incorporate acoustic output data consistent with present conventional measurement methodology.

Given the complications involved in making biophysical endpoint predictions, the validity and appropriateness of the models used for the indices remain to be tested adequately and discussed. The implications of the thermal models are summarized later in this chapter; the models provide new insight as to where and under which circumstances maximum thermal rises are to be expected.

CLINICAL APPLICATIONS

Tissue Types

For each ultrasound image or mode, ultrasound passes through several tissue or fluid layers having different acoustic and attenuation characteristics. Detailed examination of the tissue geometry of popular imaging

views for different applications, especially those involving sensitive sites, is warranted. Some work has already been performed on characteristics of the abdominal wall for fetal examinations.[3,7] These studies have a statistical component to account for variations in a population.

Because ultrasound-induced heating is proportional to the ultrasound attenuation coefficient of the insonified tissue, it is helpful to categorize tissues by their attenuation characteristics. At one extreme is bone, which is strongly attenuating; at the other extreme are fluids such as urine and amniotic fluid, which are minimally attenuating. Soft tissue on the average has an attenuation coefficient of 0.5 dB/MHz-cm. One approach frequently used in tissue modeling[5] is to use an overall conservative tissue attenuation value of 0.3 dB/MHz-cm. Although simplistic, this approximation allows a first-order estimate of tissue attenuation for heating prediction. More detailed and accurate modeling of tissue attenuation is under development.[7]

Biologically Sensitive Sites

Many sites and imaging applications have been identified as being of concern[1-3,5-8] for the potential for possible ultrasound-induced bioeffects. The most well known and important is the examination of the fetus. The embryo is particularly sensitive during the first trimester during the period of organogenesis. The temperature elevation is highest, however, in the second and third trimesters because of the presence of fetal bone. The main concern here is the possibility of damage to central nervous system structures (brain and spinal cord) adjacent to heated bone. Furthermore, because of the small attenuation in traversing amniotic fluid, there is the potential for cavitation in the vicinity of the fetus. Although these effects have never been observed to occur in diagnostic examinations, they do represent what we believe to be the most important events to watch for.

Neonatal and adult transcranial examinations are of concern because of the possibility that brain tissue might be damaged if the temperature of adjacent bone is elevated significantly. In adult transcranial applications, the ultrasound intensity is especially high to penetrate through the highly attenuating skull bone, and the temperature elevation near the bone surface may be significant.

The eye is a biologically sensitive site for ultrasound. The lens has no blood supply and thus is limited in its ability to dissipate heat. Cataract formation is possible if the lens is exposed to ultrasound intensities greater than 100 mW/cm^2 for extended periods. The retina is of concern because the vitreous and aqueous humors of the eye provide a low attenuation path for sound reaching it in ophthalmic applications. Retinal burns can be seen in high-intensity therapeutic applications.

Other areas of concern include intracavitary applications (e.g., transesophageal, intraoperative, endovaginal, and rectal) in which the transducer probe is located adjacent to or in close proximity with thermally sensitive tissues. The skin is a superb thermal barrier; its perfusion length is a mere 2 mm. By being able to maintain a large thermal gradient, the skin permits the internal temperature of the body to remain relatively constant even though the external temperature may vary over a wide range. By bypassing the skin, intracavitary applications may expose thermally sensitive tissues to the heated surface of a transducer. Self-heating results because modern pulsed transducers convert only about 10 percent of the electrical energy into acoustic energy; the remainder is largely converted into heat. Of all the potential adverse effects, thermal damage caused by self-heat-

ing of transducers is the most likely to occur in intracavitary applications.

As an example of how safety considerations can affect equipment design of an intracavitary probe, consider the special features incorporated in a particular diagnostic system using transesophageal probes. A temperature sensor is imbedded in the distal end of each transesophageal probe to aid the clinician in preventing the potential burning of esophageal tissue caused by self-heating of the transducer. The probe surface temperature is a function of both the sensor and internal patient temperatures. The probe surface temperature and a constant (not sensed) normal patient temperature of 37°C are displayed continuously by default. In the case of multiple array probes such as biplane transesophageal units, the temperature of each probe is displayed continually. The physician has the option to enter a higher patient temperature constant for a febrile patient or a lower constant for an hypothermic patient. This information is used in calculating the probe temperature at its outer surface (the hottest part of the transducer) and in determining when to issue warnings to the physician.

The computed transducer probe surface temperature is compared continually with two threshold levels (not accessible to the user). When the probe temperature exceeds the lower of the two thresholds, an appropriate warning is issued to the user. He or she may then reduce the power or make any corrections for the body temperature of the patient. If the probe temperature exceeds the second (higher) threshold, a warning is shown, power to the transducer is interrupted, and the image is frozen. The probe temperature must fall below the high threshold, either naturally or through the physician's actions, before imaging can resume. The importance of exposure time at higher temperatures is emphasized in the user's manual for the probe. As an additional safeguard, a separate hardware circuit provides redundant safety. If the upper threshold is exceeded by 1°C, ultrasound transmission is shut down and an error message is shown.

Nonlinear Heating Effects

Pressure waves from diagnostic ultrasound exhibit finite amplitude or nonlinear distortion effects in water. These effects are far less pronounced in tissue because of tissue attenuation, but they may be significant near a focus in low-loss fluids. Near a focus, enhanced heating of a sensitive tissue could occur because of the harmonic rich content of nonlinearly distorted beams; these effects are under study. Under worst-case conditions, the maximum heating enhancement is estimated to be less than a factor of 2.[2]

Diagnostic Equipment Modes

Instrument modes fall into two general types: scanned (B-mode imaging and color-flow imaging) and unscanned (stationary); and M-mode and Doppler. Combination modes may include different types of modes together. B-mode imaging is judged to be harmless insofar as heating effects go.[1,2,5] Unscanned modes provide more bioeffect risk potential.

GUIDELINES

There are two general methods for the safe and effective use of diagnostic ultrasound. The first is based on the availability of real-time thermal and mechanical (cavitation) indices.[5] The second approach, similar to that of the AIUM/NEMA output display group, is applicable when bioeffect feedback is not provided to the user.

Real-Time Output Display Approach

Figure 12-1 shows a flow chart indicating how a physician or sonographer should approach clinical decision making regarding safety in diagnostic ultrasound examinations. First, the examination should be performed only when there is some expectation of medical benefit for the patient. The next step requires an estimate of the maximum temperature elevation that could occur anywhere in the path of the ultrasound within the patient. This should be a "reasonable worst case" estimate, implying that any higher temperature would be unlikely. The clinical user would need to specify the type of examination but would need to rely on the ultrasound instrument manufacturer to provide the quantitative estimate of the maximum temperature rise for that application. This estimate, called the *thermal index* (TI), has to be updated and made available to the user whenever the ultrasound console controls are changed. The computation of the TI should be performed using the most appropriate and accurate tissue models available for the given application.

If the estimated value of the TI exceeds the value 2 (i.e., when the calculated temperature elevation exceeds 2°C), it becomes necessary to consider the duration that any anatomic structure will be exposed to the ultrasound beam. Based on the temperature versus exposure duration relationship and known bioeffect thresholds,[8] examinations lasting less than $4^{(6-TI)}$ minutes in afebrile patients may be considered "safe." Where this duration will be exceeded, it is necessary to consider possible mitigating factors when evaluating the risk/benefit ratio. Mitigating factors include the obesity and physical size of the patient, the structures being exposed, the degree of perfusion, and the presence or absence of any specially sensitive anatomic structure. If the risks of the examination exceed the anticipated benefits, either the ultrasound power should be reduced to lessen

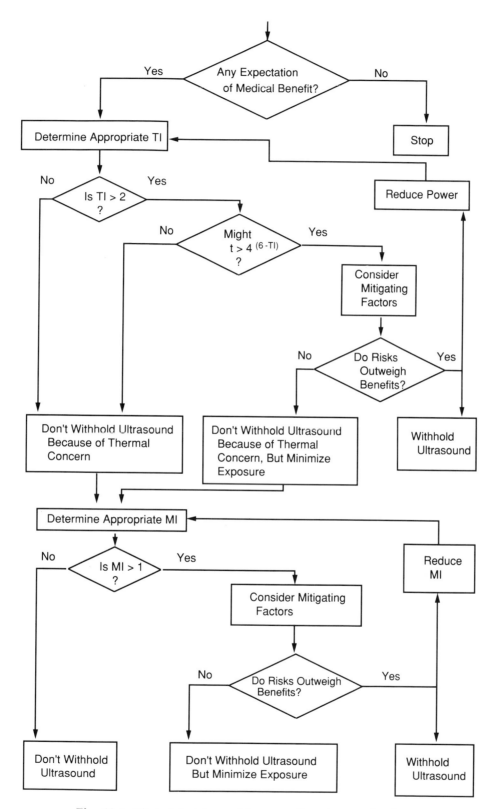

Fig. 12-1 Clinical decision making regarding ultrasound safety.

the TI or the examination should be cancelled.

After consideration of an adverse effect caused by a thermal mechanism, consideration is given to the possibility of an adverse effect arising from a mechanical effect such as transient cavitation. Here, the appropriate estimate for the likelihood of a mechanical event, the mechanical index (MI), needs to be made available to the user by the ultrasound manufacturer, using the best available physical and tissue models. In this case, the MI versus exposure duration relationship has not yet been developed. Otherwise, the logic in the flow diagram follows that given for thermal concerns.

Relative ALARA Approach in the Absence of Real-Time Output Display

Although the information presented here is complementary to that in the previous section, there is no information of a specific bioeffects nature assumed to be provided to the user (other than possibly an equipment class rating). As a start, the application and intended imaging view is considered.

1. Does the application include sensitive sites; if so, where in the image are they located?

2. What does the acoustic path to the site include in terms of soft tissue, fluid, or bone?

3. What characteristics of the person being imaged differ from the norm: thin or heavy, healthy, body type, age, and so on? Does the ultrasound mode include a nonscanning modality? If so, the mode should be considered nonscanning.

4. What transducer is to be used? What are the aperture dimensions and area, center frequency, fixed focal length (focus) if any, and intended adjustable focus of the transducer?

5. What controls on the instrument affect acoustic output? Is there a separate transmit or output control?

6. The above information can be used with the chart in Table 12-1 to estimate where maximum heating or cavitation could potentially occur. This information can be applied in conjunction with the user's knowledge of the location of the sensitive site. Columns (increase/decrease) in the chart indicate how the bioeffects depend directly on parameters within the user's control (items 4 and 5), and also on related physical quantities shown in parentheses in the table.

7. The ALARA principle should be used. Knowledge of system operation should be used to apply ALARA. Of special interest are the controls that affect the peak output and power in nonscanning modes.

Trends in Modern Diagnostic Imaging Equipment

Newer imaging systems are growing in complexity to offer clinicians improved performance, new modalities, capabilities, and applications. As a result of these changes, it is becoming increasingly difficult for users of the equipment to be sure which controls affect acoustic output without feedback indicators based on the actual operation of the system. This complexity is a consequence of the interrelationship of many factors[6] (scan depth, pulse repetition rate, and so on), internally applied limits to output (regulatory ceilings on different output parameters, surface temperature limits, design advantages, and so on), and equipment limitations (power supply limits, design shortfalls, boundaries, and so on).

Simplistic viewpoints regarding acoustic output apply only to the most basic equipment. Without a prior knowledge of equipment design, it is often difficult for a user to know how to affect acoustic output even though he or she may be proficient in using the instrument. For example, as a general rule, receiver gain controls should be used in conjunction with transmit or acoustic output level controls to minimize output and to ob-

Table 12-1 Conditions Affecting the Potential for Bioeffects

Bioeffect Type	Clinical Application	Mode	Transducer Aperture Area	Location of Maximum	Increase With	Decrease With
Thermal	Soft tissue	Scan	Any	Surface	Power, frequency	
	Soft tissue	No scan	Large, >1 cm^2	Intermediate, <focus	Power, (ISPTA), frequency	Depth, (attenuation)
	Soft tissue	No scan	Small, <1 cm^2	Surface	Power, frequency	
	Soft tissue/bone	Scan	Any	Surface	Power, frequency	
	Bone at focus	No scan	Any	Focus	Aperture size, frequency	Focus, (depth), focal beam width
	Bone at surface	Scan/no scan	Any	Surface	Power	Aperture size
Cavitation	Soft tissue	Any	Any	Intermediate, <focus	(Peak pressure amplitude), transmit level	Square root of frequency, depth, (attenuation)
	Fluid path	Any	Any	Focus	(Peak pressure amplitude), transmit level	Square root of frequency

tain diagnostic information of acceptable quality. On some equipment, the receiver gain and transmit output are locked together with limited adjustment available to the user. As a general rule, the increase in pulse repetition rate over a given region for a combination mode compared with a B-mode image of the same size and format is roughly inversely proportional to the factor by which the frame rate decreases. This rule assumes that an accurate display of frame rate is available, but there are exceptions. If a system is designed to deliver constant output power in Doppler modes, pressure amplitude and repetition rates are inversely rated; however, this design information is usually unknown to the user. Therefore, without real-time display of thermal and mechanical indices, it is difficult to implement the ALARA principle meaningfully on a specific imaging system. Given the complex operation of modern diagnostic imaging systems, it is necessary for the clinician to have this relevant indication of bioeffect potential at the time of an examination to minimize risk to the patient.

REFERENCES

1. Docker MF, Duck FA (eds): The Safe Use of Diagnostic Ultrasound. British Medical Ultrasound Society/British Institute of Radiology, London, 1991

2. World Federation for Ultrasound in Medicine and Biology: Issues and recommendations regarding thermal mechanisms for biological effects of ultrasound. Ultrasound Med Biol 18: 731, 1992

3. National Council on Radiation Protection and Measurements: Biological Effects of Ultrasound: Mechanisms and Clinical Implications. Report 74. NCRP, Bethesda, Maryland, 1983

4. Apfel RE, Holland CK: Gauging the likelihood of cavitation from short pulse, low duty-cycle diagnostic ultrasound. Ultrasound Med Biol 17:179, 1991

5. American Institute of Ultrasound in Medicine/National Electrical Manufacturers' Association: Standard for Realtime Display of Thermal and Mechanical Indices on Diagnostic Ultrasound Equipment. AIUM, Rockville, Maryland, 1992

6. Szabo TL, Melton HE, Hempstead PS: Ultrasonic output measurements of multiple-mode diagnostic ultrasound systems. IEEE Trans Ultrason Ferroelect Freq Contr 35:220, 1988

7. National Council on Radiation Protection and Measurements: Exposure Criteria for Medical Diagnostic Ultrasound: 1. Criteria Based on Thermal Mechanisms. Report 113. NCRP, Bethesda, Maryland, 1992

8. Miller MW, Ziskin MC: Biological consequences of hyperthermia. Ultrasound Med Biol 15:707, 1989

13

Quality Management of Ultrasound Diagnosis

Michael F. Insana
Timothy J. Hall

Quality management of diagnostic ultrasound equipment has traditionally focused on acceptance testing and routine quality assurance testing. Acceptance testing, which for some is a contingency of the purchase, ensures that the system performs according to the specifications that attracted the buyer in the first place. With acceptance testing procedures, we assume that the diagnostic quality of the image produced can be assessed through measurements of essential engineering properties of the system. There are standards to guide those performing acceptance testing procedures.[1] These standards rarely specify acceptable results, in part because acceptable levels for image quality are task-specific (e.g., spatial resolution is more critical than gray-scale resolution for echocardiography whereas the opposite is often true for abdominal ultrasound). The greatest value of acceptance testing procedures has been to set a level of performance for later comparisons

in a quality assurance program. The function of quality assurance testing is to document degradations in image quality over time. If important features of image quality are monitored carefully and routinely, the service agreements that manufacturers provide can be used effectively to maintain high standards of image quality as well as to correct catastrophic failures.

Careful monitoring of image quality has been an important element in providing the highest quality diagnostic examination. Until recently, analog electronic components—characteristically fast but likely to produce drifting signal strengths—were used to form and display real-time images. Manufacturers are now substituting digital components for their analog counterparts to increase the quality and stability of imaging for less cost. In addition, microprocessors are used frequently to measure automatically the performance of essential subsystems, to report to the user any substandard results, and to help to identify sources of error to service personnel. These developments have led some people to question the need for a rigorous quality assurance program in diagnostic ultrasound. At the same time, the proliferation of speciality transducer probes designed for specific clinical applications emphasizes the need for acceptance testing to determine imaging properties and hence the advantages and disadvantages of each probe. This evolution in imaging systems has brought about a new goal for acceptance testing—which is to measure those transducer properties that determine image quality so that users can choose the most appropriate probe for each examination. This choice requires that the trade-offs in image quality intended by manufacturers for each probe design should be interpreted for clinical imaging objectives. For example, in situations where the footprint size is not a significant factor, what losses in image quality can be expected using a phased array instead of a linear array, and how do those losses affect diagnostic performance?

As many of the more mundane issues of instrumentation performance are solved by advances in electronics and engineering and as the dazzling array of probe designs and imaging options continues to expand, we believe that the proper choice of probe and image processing become the limiting factors in image quality management. Manufacturers of high-end radiology products are moving away from systems that specialize in one clinical area and toward systems that can encompass a broad range of examinations but with probes specially designed for specific examinations. Thus, to obtain the highest possible image quality, users must understand the basic engineering properties of each probe design in terms of image quality and interpret that information for each clinical task. Unlike previous approaches to this subject, our method attempts to define image

quality to relate engineering properties of systems to image detectability, using graphic rather than mathematic examples to show how the limitations of probe designs affect the detectability of targets in the image. We also explore methods for estimating image quality parameters that may be used in acceptance testing procedures.

IMAGE QUALITY

The quality of an image is easier to recognize than to define. The highest-quality images are shown in the manufacturers' advertisements in most journals. Although the quality of the image depends directly on the imaging system, the diagnostic value of the examination, which we call *target detectability*, depends on the properties of the tissues imaged, the skill of the operator, and the quality of the display, in addition to image quality (Fig. 13-1). Such "targets" as focal lesions, cysts, and blood vessels can be broadly classified for image quality purposes in their size, contrast, and surface reflectivity, as we discuss later. Some of the less common and more narrow terms are defined in Table 13-1.

Image quality is defined in terms of the quality and uniformity of spatial resolution and gray-scale resolution. Both types of resolutions are often measured from beam profiles that are characteristic of the entire system but in particular the transducer (e.g., Fig. 13-2). The beamwidth in the image plane determines lateral resolution, and the beamwidth perpendicular to the image plane determines elevational resolution. The transmitted pulse length and receiver bandwidth determine axial resolution.

Spatial resolution refers to the ability of the system to display closely positioned structures as discrete targets (Fig. 13-3A). The half amplitude (-6 dB) or one-tenth amplitude (-20 dB) beamwidths characterize spatial

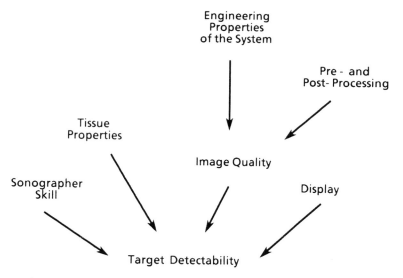

Fig. 13-1 Outline of components of target detectability and image.

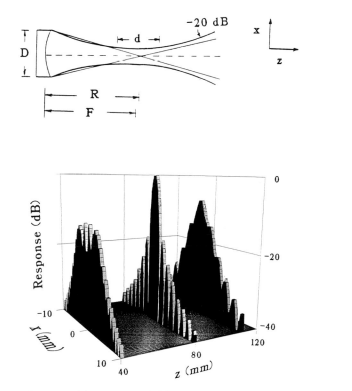

Fig. 13-2 (Top) Long-axis view of the pressure field from a circular, spherically focused, piezoelectric element of diameter D. R, radius of curvature; F, focal length; and d, depth of focus. **(Bottom)** Three lateral beam profiles simulated in water (20 degrees C) assuming D = 19 mm, R = 80 mm, and the resonant frequency is 5 MHz.

Table 13-1 Definitions

Array channels	Electronic pulse-receiver pairs in the beam former that are connected to transducer array elements to transmit pulses and receive echoes; independent channels perform without cross-talk
Apodization	Unequal weighting given to signals on array elements to reduce grating lobe amplitudes at the expense of increasing the width of the main lobe
Beam former	Electronic components that transmit, delay, and sum signals from array channels to form, focus, and steer the sound beam
Beam profiles	How the amplitude of the pressure field varies with position in the field
Contrast	Many definitions. *Object contrast* is the difference between backscatter coefficients for the target and background divided by that of the background. Object contrast is a function of frequency. *Target contrast* is similar, except that the backscatter coefficients are weighted and summed over the frequency response of the system and over the volume interrogated by the beam. *Image contrast* includes those features of target contrast and any postprocessing of the image. Target contrast and image contrast are frequency independent
Dynamic range	Ratio of the smallest echo amplitude that just saturates the display to the smallest echo amplitude that produces a signal on the display at the threshold of detection
f-number	Ratio of the focal length to the aperture size; low *f*-number transducers (e.g., 2 or less) are considered strongly focused
Focal length	Axial distance between the piezoelectric element(s) and field point with maximum acoustic intensity; the focal length varies with frequency and sound speed, whereas the radius of curvature does not
Focal region	Volume in the pressure field centered near the focal length whose axial dimension is determined by the transducer depth of field
Footprint	Surface area of the transducer that contacts the patient's skin
High-contrast gray-scale resolution	Ability of the system to display regions of different but similar reflectivities as discrete regions, in a mixed field of strong and weak reflectors
Image quality	Quality and uniformity of spatial and gray-scale resolutions
Low-contrast resolution	Ability of the system to display gray-scale regions of different but similar reflectivities as discrete regions
Partial volume	When scattered signals from structures outside image plane are mispositioned in the image plane; the principal cause in ultrasound is poor elevational resolution. Partial volume effects reduce target contrast
Radius of curvature	Fixed point in space determined by the curvature of the piezoelectric elements or lens
Sensitivity	Smallest echo amplitude that produces a signal on the display at the threshold of detection; together the sensitivity and dynamic range specify the detectable range of echo signals
Spatial resolution	Ability of the system to display closely positioned structures as discrete targets; spatial resolution is specified in three dimensions as axial, lateral (also called *azimuthal*), and elevational
Transducer aperture	Length or area of piezoelectric material that transmits or receives acoustic energy; for resolution, the effective aperture can vary with steering angle and apodization

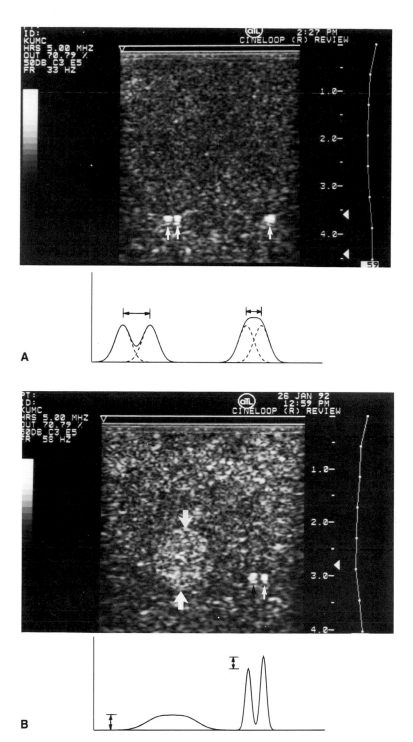

Fig. 13-3 Examples of spatial and gray-scale resolution using a linear array. Large arrows indicate location of targets. **(A)** Spatial resolution: four nylon wires, 0.36 mm in diameter, imaged through a cross-sectional plane. Left pair are resolvable as distinct targets, but right pair are not. Arrows in graph indicate interval separation of peak signal strength. **(B)** Gray-scale resolution: 12-mm-diameter target on left is slightly more echogenic than the background. This is an example of an imaging task that requires superior low-contrast gray-scale resolution. If, in the same image, we also wish to detect the change in reflectivity of the two nylon wires on the right (0.30-mm and 0.36-mm diameters), we require that the imaging system should have superior high-contrast gray-scale resolution. Arrows in graph indicate separation and magnitude of peak signal strength.

resolution. The -20-dB beamwidth is sometimes chosen because it corresponds to roughly the half brightness level on the video display.[2] Often the axial spatial resolution is constant throughout the field and superior to the lateral spatial resolution, which varies with depth (z-axis). When the lateral beamwidth is approximately equal to the pulse duration, the axial and lateral spatial resolutions are equal so that point targets appear as round dots rather than arcs.

Gray-scale resolution refers to the ability of the system to display regions of similar reflectivity as discrete regions (low-contrast gray-scale resolution), as well as to differentiate structures of similar reflectivity in a mixed field of strong and weak reflectors (high-contrast gray-scale resolution) (Fig. 13-3B). Gray-scale resolution is degraded by clutter from mispositioned, low-amplitude echoes produced by off-axis beam energy. This is similar to the degradation of radiograph image contrast from Compton scattering in the body. The elevational beamwidth and the -40-dB to -60-dB lateral beamwidths, corresponding to the lowest-amplitude echoes, determine the gray-scale resolution of the system.

Finally, a large dynamic range always improves image quality, particularly high-contrast gray-scale resolution, but the effects of high sensitivity depend on the beam profile. High sensitivity makes it possible to image low-amplitude target echoes. If there is a broad -40-dB bandwidth, however, sensitivity to low-amplitude echoes can also reduce low-contrast gray-scale resolution. Statements regarding image quality involve a complex interaction between resolution, sensitivity, and dynamic range. To maximize target detectability, an operator must choose the transducer that emphasizes the elements of image quality necessary to reach specific diagnostic goals.

This definition of image quality is for a single image and ignores the important real-time features of ultrasound. Conspicuously missing from our definition of image quality are line density and frame rate. We believe that because the selection of both features is determined by the diagnostic goals of the examination and ultimately by the speed of sound in tissues, these parameters are not fundamental to image quality but rather tools to be used to maximize detectability. Therefore, these features influence detectability through the operator skill component identified in Figure 13-1.

FIXED-FOCUS TRANSDUCERS

The three lateral beam profiles in Figure 13-2 illustrate the kinds of variations in image quality characteristics of fixed-focus, mechanical sector probes. Near the radius of curvature ($z = 80$ mm), acoustic energy is concentrated in a narrow main lobe with little energy in the side lobes. Hence, the focal region produces the highest sensitivity and resolution, both spatial and gray scale. The elevational and lateral beamwidths are equal for circularly symmetric, piezoelectric elements. A large aperture size gives a narrow main lobe and high sensitivity near the radius of curvature where resolution is greatest.

Fixed-focus transducers cannot yield high image quality over a large field of view, because the resolution is characteristically nonuniform. In the far-field ($z = 220$ mm in Fig. 13-2), the peak pressure is reduced, the main lobe broadens, and the side lobe pressure increases relative to the main lobe. Near the radius of curvature and in the far-field, the speckle spot size is a good indicator of spatial resolution.[3] In the near-field ($z = 40$ mm), distinctions between main and side lobes are lost. The multiple peaks in the near-field beam profile produce fine image texture (i.e., small speckle spots), giving a false impression of high spatial resolution. In terms of the ability to resolve closely spaced targets (Fig. 13-3A), the spatial resolution in the near-field is very poor although the image texture is very fine.

Axial spatial resolution remains essentially constant throughout the field. The short transmit pulse duration needed for high axial spatial resolution reduces sensitivity. Narrowband pulses increase sensitivity but decrease axial spatial resolution.

ARRAY TRANSDUCERS

The principal advantage of arrays over fixed-focus transducers is their ability to produce uniform resolution in the image plane throughout the field of view and hence to give higher image quality. Fixed-focus transducers can give very high resolution over a limited region, which is important for some clinical examinations, but the definition of image quality already given states that the quality *and* uniformity of resolution are essential features of high-quality images. Specific clinical applications determine the need for each type of probe.

As with the fixed-focus probes, large aperture arrays yield high spatial resolution and sensitivity in media with homogeneous sound velocity. The aperture size (D) and wavelength of sound (λ) at the resonant frequency determine the width of the main lobe (Fig. 13-4A and B). Element spacing (d) and λ determine the position of the grating lobes. The width of the elements (w), axial position (z), and λ control the directivity for an element (the dashed lines in Fig. 13-4B and C).[4] The element directivity function weights the directivity for the array (solid lines in Fig. 13-4B and C), such that when the elements are spaced $\lambda/2$ apart, grating lobes are minimized because the grating lobes are positioned near the zeroes of the element directivity. In addition, elements must be connected to separate and yet matched electronic channels that transmit and receive signals independently of each other. Manufacturers construct arrays with as many channels as possible, as determined primarily by the cost the market will bear.

The independently controlled elements give arrays the flexibility needed for high quality and uniform resolution. For example, the beam profile for transmitting pulses can be different from the beam profile for receiving echoes. The principles involved are that the lateral and elevational spatial resolutions are given by the products of their respective transmit and receive beam profiles.[5] (Transmit and receive beam profiles are the same in elevation for one-dimensional arrays because arrays are mechanically focused in elevation and therefore operate as fixed-focus transducers.) Array pulse sequences are designed to transmit a number of pulses per image line equal to the number of transmit foci selected. Consequently, the frame rate decreases as the number of transmit zones is increased. Signals are dynamically focused on receive by systematically delaying the reception of echo signals on each channel (Fig. 13-4A) before summation and envelope detection. The aperture grows (i.e., the number of active piezoelectric elements increases) as the focal length increases to maintain a constant f-number. A constant f-number is necessary to obtain uniform image plane resolution throughout the field. This look-forward beam forming process is typical of linear array transducers, which have large footprints that require ample access to target organs. Curved linear arrays have smaller footprints and uniformly high image plane resolution, similar to linear arrays, except that the degree of curvature often limits the maximum aperture size. Therefore, the spatial resolution for curved linear arrays is sometimes lower than that for linear arrays.

Phased arrays focus and steer the beam electronically. This feature greatly reduces the

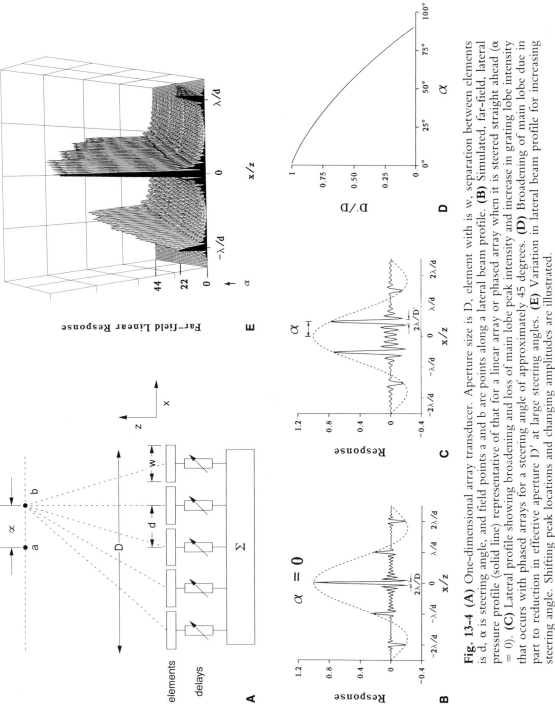

Fig. 13-4 (A) One-dimensional array transducer. Aperture size is D, element with is w, separation between elements is d, α is steering angle, and field points a and b are points along a lateral beam profile. **(B)** Simulated, far-field, lateral pressure profile (solid line) representative of that for a linear array or phased array when it is steered straight ahead (α = 0). **(C)** Lateral profile showing broadening and loss of main lobe peak intensity and increase in grating lobe intensity that occurs with phased arrays for a steering angle of approximately 45 degrees. **(D)** Broadening of main lobe due in part to reduction in effective aperture D' at large steering angles. **(E)** Variation in lateral beam profile for increasing steering angle. Shifting peak locations and changing amplitudes are illustrated.

footprint without necessarily reducing the aperture. Phased arrays provide easy access to many hard-to-reach regions (e.g., the heart). Unfortunately, beam steering reduces all aspects of image quality at large steering angles in comparison with linear arrays. A graphic representation of the changes in beam profile that occur when the beam is steered from point *a* to point *b* (Fig. 13-4A), over the sector angle α, may be seen in Figure 13-4B and C. Steering the beam to the right, through an angle α, is equivalent to "sliding" the array directivity (solid lines) to the right with respect to the element directivity (dashed lines). There are two principal consequences of beam steering on resolution and sensitivity (Fig. 13-4E). First, the amplitude of the main lobe decreases while that of the first side lobe increases because of the way in which these peaks are weighted by the element directivity (dashed lines in Fig. 13-4B and C). As a result, gray-scale resolution and sensitivity decrease at large steering angles. Second, the effective aperture size D' (the

projection of D on a line perpendicular to the line of sight) is reduced for increasing α (Fig. 13-4D), which has the effect of broadening the main lobe and reducing lateral spatial resolution. Compare the main lobe widths for the pressure profiles in Figure 13-4B and C, where α = 0 and α = 45 degrees, respectively. Between these two angles, the lateral beam profile varies with steering angle as shown in Figure 13-4E. Beam steering of linear arrays sometimes is used in Doppler applications. In this situation, the Doppler signal from a linear array can suffer the same loss of sensitivity and resolution as a phased array used for B-mode imaging.

One commonly used method for reducing prominent grating lobes at large steering angles is apodization—an amplitude weighting of the transmit or receive signals, or both, so that elements near the center of the aperture are given more weight than those near the edge. Apodization suppresses grating lobes but also broadens the main lobe. Therefore

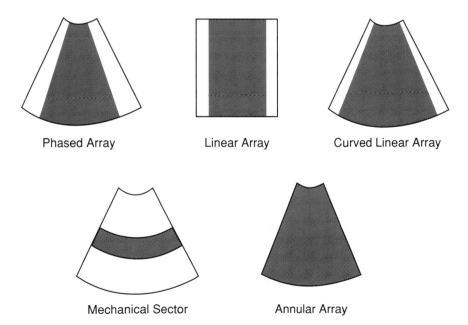

Phased Array   Linear Array   Curved Linear Array

Mechanical Sector   Annular Array

Fig. 13-5 Shaded areas illustrate regions of high lateral spatial resolution and gray-scale resolution for five different transducer designs. We assume that multiple focus on transmit and dynamic focus on receive are used with all arrays. Elevation resolution is ignored.

Table 13-2 Engineering Properties That Affect Image Quality

Engineering Property	Effect on Image Quality
Size and growth of transmit and receive apertures	Large aperture size yields superior lateral spatial resolution. Variable aperture size enables f-number to remain constant with depth to provide uniform spatial resolution
Number and position of transmit zones	Provides uniformly high spatial resolution throughout the region of interest
Number, size and spacing of piezoelectric elements; number of independent array channels	In the image plane: spacing elements one-half the resonant frequency wavelength suppresses grating lobes and increases gray-scale resolution. Where size is approximately equal to spacing and the number is large, sensitivity is maximum. Large number of elements on independent electronic channels gives high spatial resolution
f-number	Small f-numbers yield high lateral spatial resolution and shallow depth of field, requiring many transmit foci to obtain uniform spatial resolution. For strongly focused transducers (low f-numbers), depth of focus is proportional to f-number^2
Transmit and receive apodization	Weighting the center elements more than the side elements (apodization) decreases grating lobe amplitude but broadens the main lobe. Therefore apodization is a method for increasing gray-scale resolution (reducing grating lobes) at the expense of spatial resolution (broad main lobe)
Transducer bandwidth and center frequency	Spatial resolution increases with frequency (shorter pulse lengths and narrower beam widths) as depth of penetration decreases because of tissue attenuation. High bandwidths increase axial spatial resolution but decrease transducer sensitivity
Receive sensitivity and dynamic range	In general, high receive sensitivity and dynamic range increase gray-scale resolution. If the beam properties are poor, however, gray-scale resolution can decrease as receive sensitivity and dynamic range increase
Output power	Increasing output power increases system sensitivity until nonlinear propagation effects begin. Nonlinear effects transfer energy to high-frequency harmonics, which are preferentially attenuated in tissue and for which the system is insensitive to receive. Image quality features are marginally increased with large increases in power[6]
Frame rate (R); line density (N); image width and depth (Z)	High frame rate is required to avoid temporal aliasing and maximize temporal information density. High line density is required to avoid spatial aliasing and maximize spatial information density. The limited speed of sound, c, dictates how these parameters are traded off according to $c = 2ZNR$ for gray-scale imaging. Similar compromises are required for Doppler applications

apodization is a method for improving gray-scale resolution at the expense of lateral spatial resolution.

An annular array is a kind of hybrid of a mechanical sector transducer and a linear array. Annular arrays offer the superior elevational spatial resolution of mechanical sector probes in the focal region with the uniform resolution of an array. Because annular arrays typically have 12 or fewer elements, they cannot maintain a constant f-number to the same extent as other arrays with 48 to 128 channels.

In summary, linear, curved linear, and annular arrays provide the most uniform resolution throughout the field but have large footprints. Fixed-focus mechanical sector transducers and phased arrays have small footprints but nonuniform resolution, although the natures of the nonuniformities are very different (Fig. 13-5). Annular arrays and fixed-focus transducers offer elevational spatial resolution comparable with the lateral resolution and are useful for avoiding partial volume effects. Of the two, annular arrays provide more uniform resolution. Linear arrays generally have the largest footprint but the highest in-plane image quality of all the transducer designs, which is why they are popular for most examinations where accessibility to tissues and elevational resolution are not controlling factors. (Breast imaging may be the exception, as described later.) Compared with linear arrays, curved linear arrays sometimes decrease the footprint at the expense of the aperture. Phased arrays provide a small footprint and all the advantages of large aperture arrays, except uniform resolution. For small steering angles, phased arrays provide high image quality and accessibility, which explains their popularity for echocardiography. The resolution is degraded significantly at larger steering angles, limiting their general use in radiology applications. Relationships between engineer-ing properties of imaging systems and image quality are summarized in Table 13-2.

TARGET DETECTABILITY

Detectability refers to the ability of an observer to discern a target as distinct from its background. For example, the reduced resolution of phased arrays at large steering angles lowers the detectability of large, low-contrast targets as compared with that at small steering angles (Fig. 13-6). Rigorously defined,[3,7] the low-contrast detectability is given by the lesion signal-to-noise ratio, SNR_1:

$$SNR_1 = SNR_0 C_1 \left(\frac{S_1}{S_c}\right)^{-1/2} \qquad (1)$$

SNR_1 is an estimate of the detectability of the signal from the lesion averaged over the lesion area and compared with the average background signal over a similar area. SNR_o is the signal-to-noise ratio for a point in the image and may be estimated by the average background signal strength divided by its standard deviation. For linear (uncompressed) B-scan images, $SNR_0 = 1.91$. Alternatively, SNR_0^{-1}—the speckle contrast or noise in the image—may be specified. C_1 is the lesion contrast given by the echogenicity of the lesion in comparison with its background. Echogenicity may refer to digital pixel values when describing image contrast or to backscatter coefficients when describing object contrast. Gray-scale resolution of the imaging system affects image and target contrast but not object contrast (Table 13-1). S_1 is the area of the lesion and S_c is the area of a speckle spot in the far-field; their ratio describes the number of independent samples per lesion available to the observer for detection.

Equation 1 provides an explanation of how the features of image quality affect lesion detectability. Many signal processing schemes

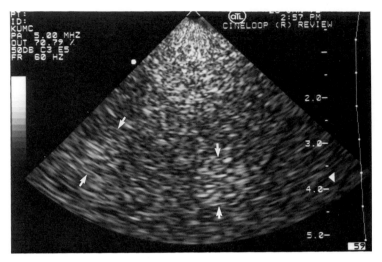

Fig. 13-6 Two identical low-contrast targets imaged using phased array and tissue-mimicking phantom material. At small steering angles (center), target is more visible than at large steering angles (left) where spatial and gray-scale resolutions are decreased. Arrows indicate location of targets.

that reduce speckle contrast (e.g., logarithmic compression) increase SNR_0 but also decrease C_1[8]: The effect on lesion detectability depends on the specific imaging task. In general, high-compression postprocessing achieves the greatest improvement in detectability when imaging high-contrast targets of all sizes, as in echocardiography. Image compounding is another speckle reduction technique, which in this case trades off spatial resolution to obtain noise reduction.[5] For this reason, compounding provides the greatest increase in detectability when the task is to detect large, low-contrast targets, because the loss of spatial resolution is less important.

It is obvious that high spatial resolution is needed to detect small targets. Equation 1 also predicts that high spatial resolution improves the detectability of large, low-contrast lesions. High spatial resolution decreases the size of the speckle spots in the image, S_c. In the far-field of the transducer, small speckle spots mean there are more independent samples per target area, which increases the information available to the observer and consequently the detectability of the target. In the near-field of the transducer, however, the speckle spots are small but not statistically independent. Therefore, the number of independent samples is not increased, and with the addition of low gray-scale resolution and high image noise, there is poor target detectability in the near-field.

Grating lobes reduce lesion detectability by decreasing target contrast. In effect, echoes from the off-axis acoustic energy in grating lobes are added to on-axis echoes, reducing the difference in reflectivity between target and background. Apodized arrays increase

Fig. 13-7 Nonscattering, 19 mm-diameter, agar wafer 1.7 mm thick imaged at three depths using a linear array to illustrate partial volume effects caused by elevational focusing. **(A)** In near-field of elevational focus, echogenicity of the target increases as the out-of-plane beamwidth increases. **(B)** Near the 35-mm elevational focal length, target is nearly echo-free because most of beam energy is focused near image plane. **(C)** In far-field, the effect is similar to that in near-field.

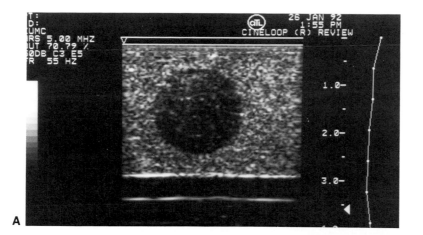

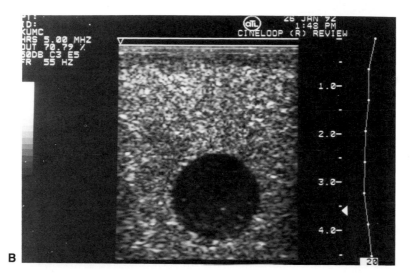

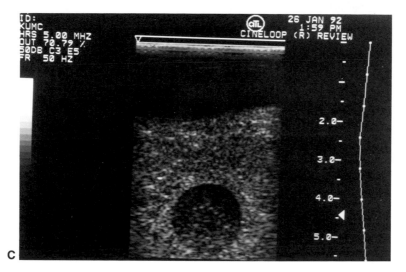

the detectability for imaging large, low-contrast targets by decreasing grating lobe amplitudes. Apodization should not be used where high spatial resolution is specifically needed. Eventually, manufacturers may provide controls to allow users to adjust the transmit and receive apodization to fit specific needs.

The spatial resolution of a transducer in elevation is not estimated as easily from the image as are lateral and axial spatial resolutions. Like grating lobes, poor elevational resolution reduces contrast by adding off-axis echoes to on-axis echoes. But in this case, the off-axis echoes are from structures located outside the image plane. Figure 13-7 is an example of the loss of contrast outside the elevational focal zone for a linear array mechanically focused in elevation at 35 mm. In all three images, a thin, nonscattering, agar disk has been carefully positioned so that the beam axis lies within the thickness of the disk. In the elevational focal zone, near a depth of 35 mm, the agar disk appears as ideally it should, nearly echo-free (Fig. 13-7B). But in the near- and far-fields (Fig. 13-7A and C), we see an increasing echogenicity that demonstrates the loss of contrast, or partial volume effects, where the beam is broad. An operator may determine whether partial volume effects are filling in an otherwise echo-free target by changing the target depth using a stand-off pad or by changing to an annular array.

The absorption and heterogeneity of body tissues impose the ultimate limitations on efforts to increase spatial resolution through higher frequencies and larger apertures. It is well known that high-frequency sound is attenuated more than low-frequency sound. Because of the frequency dependence of attenuation, the operator, wishing to optimize detectability, selects a probe with a center frequency appropriate for the examination based on the need to balance sensitivity and spatial resolution (e.g., low-frequency trans-

ducers are used to increase the sensitivity for imaging deep in the body at the expense of spatial resolution). Similarly, highly heterogeneous tissues such as fatty breasts require smaller apertures than other structures to maximize detectability. Irregularly shaped boundaries between media with different speeds of sound, such as those between fat and glandular tissues in the breast, distort the coherent wavefronts passing through the boundary, defocusing the beam.[9,10] Wavefront aberrations shift main lobe energy off-axis, decreasing both spatial and gray-scale resolutions. Large apertures pass acoustic energy through large superficial body areas and therefore are more likely to suffer wavefront distortions. In abdominal imaging, body wall layers are more planar and therefore less aberrating, so that large apertures yield greater detectability. Consequently, tissue heterogeneity should influence the selection of transducer aperture as attenuation does transducer frequency.

In summary, aperture size, f-number, and resonance frequency are the principal factors determining spatial resolution. The type of transducer, amount of apodization, and position of the target in the field are principal factors determining gray-scale resolution. These are the features that must be considered when selecting a transducer for an examination. Methods of measuring these and other features for acceptance testing are described in the next section.

ACCEPTANCE TESTING METHODS

There are various measurement techniques for evaluating image quality using ultrasound test objects and laboratory equipment. These methods include tests applicable to gray-scale imaging and those intended to evaluate flow measurements. Only those tests applicable to both mechanical sector and array transducers are discussed.

Equipment

TEST OBJECTS

Many test objects for evaluating different aspects of ultrasound imaging devices are commercially available. The best known is the AIUM 100-mm test object (Nuclear Associates, Carle Place, New York), which was designed to measure axial and lateral resolution, dead zone, registration, and range accuracy. Other more versatile test objects, such as the RMI 415 (Radiation Measurements Inc., Middleton, Wisconsin) or the ATS 519 (ATS Laboratories Inc., Bridgeport, Connecticut), contain tissue-mimicking (TM) hydrogel media that have acoustic attenuation, scattering, and sound speed similar to those of human liver. TM test objects are often referred to as *phantoms*. Other test objects designed for evaluation of flow measurement devices and special applications (transvaginal, transrectal, etc.) are also available. Phantoms are essential for routine quality assurance programs because they provide summary measures of important image quality features under clinical conditions that can be tracked over time. Often acceptance testing procedures require more detailed analyses and specialized laboratory equipment.

LABORATORY EQUIPMENT

Beam profiles are central to the evaluation of image quality. Standard equipment for measuring beam profiles directly includes a hydrophone (very small aperture transducer), a three-dimensional positioning device, temperature-controlled water container, function generator, and waveform digitizer.

Several types of hydrophones are available from many manufacturers (e.g., Specialty Engineering Associates, Milpitas, California, and NTR Systems Inc., Seattle, Washington). Typically, the single piezoelectric element in hydrophones commonly used for diagnostic ultrasound is a material (polyvinylidene difluoride) known as *PVDF*. The resonant frequency of PVDF is typically 25 MHz or higher, resulting in a fairly flat frequency response at diagnostic frequencies. Apertures as small as 0.2 mm provide minimal spatial averaging, which is important for mapping beam profiles.

Positioning devices are used systematically to map pressure fields. Most of these devices are custom-made from standard optics equipment, but some fully configured devices such as that by Panametrics (Panametrics Inc., Waltham, Massachusetts) and NTR (NTR Systems Inc., Seattle, Washington) are available. Acoustic output is measured in distilled and degassed water that is temperature-controlled to maintain constant propagation speed of the acoustic pulses.

To determine the system's response during reception independent of the transmission properties, a function generator is used to transmit known signals. High stability in signal amplitude, frequency, and phase for the function generator are extremely important. High-speed transient recorders, such as digital oscilloscopes, are used to record and display waveforms.

The equipment just described can provide a detailed assessment of image quality directly but also requires a significant investment of time and money. Many of the procedures described later measure beam properties indirectly, using test objects wherever possible to obtain summary measures of image quality.

GRAY-SCALE IMAGING

To assess image quality, we wish to measure those parameters that affect the quality and uniformity of the spatial and gray-scale resolutions. A logical first step is to verify the accurate mapping of acoustic data to the image, or registration accuracy and measurement calibration. A logical second step is to determine the axial range over which data can be acquired. This range is limited in the near-field by the ringdown distance of the transducer and in the far-field by the maximum depth of penetration. Related parameters are the acoustic output, sensitivity, and dynamic range of the system. Subsequent tests include evaluation of spatial resolution, spectral response, and transmit and receive apertures. Finally, the quality and uniformity of the photographic system must be tested.

Registration Accuracy and Measurement Calibration

Calibration of depth markers and electronic calipers and verification of registration accuracy can be performed by scanning a TM test object and measuring the displayed separation between targets[1] (Fig. 13-8A). In this RMI phantom, the horizontal and vertical rows of nylon line targets are spaced 3 cm and 2 cm, respectively. Once calibrated, calipers and depth markers can be used confidently in the following tests.

Ringdown Distance

Ringdown distance is the distance from the top of the image along the beam axis to the first identifiable echo that is free from multiple reflections. The ringdown distance is greater than or equal to the dead zone interval, which is the axial distance to the first identifiable echo. Both quantities are measured using a TM test object and depth markers or calipers. The images in Figure 13-7 show a negligible dead zone but a significant ringdown distance extending approximately 4 mm from the transducer face. Minimal ringdown distance is important, particularly in peripheral vascular imaging.

Depth of Penetration

Penetration is generally measured by scanning a TM test object with the system output and far-field gain set to maximum levels and measuring the depth at which echo signals from the background medium are displayed just above electronic noise levels (Fig. 13-8A). Penetration varies with system output, tissue attenuation, and echogenicity, as well as with the sensitivity and gain of the receiver. Therefore, phantoms used to measure penetration must be well characterized. Alternatively, penetration can be estimated from two system-dependent measurements: system output and receiver sensitivity. In the United States, federal regulations specify the methods for measuring system output[11] and currently limit its value. Receiver sensitivity for the system can be measured independently of transmission properties by receiving signals from a hydrophone used as a transmitter and located in a water tank near the transducer focal position. With system output minimized and receiver gain maximized, continuous-wave (CW) signals are generated with the hydrophone at the resonance frequency of the transducer. The amplitude of the CW signal is reduced until the detected signal just disappears in the image noise. That amplitude is a measure of receiver sensitivity. A less subjective measure is to view the video signal on an oscilloscope and to determine the amplitude of the CW signal required to create a television signal just above the noise level. Hydrophone calibration allows conversion from the minimum voltage driving the hydrophone to the minimum detectable pressure by the transducer. Typically, electronic noise limits sensitivity on high-end ultrasound scanners.

System Dynamic Range

As defined above, dynamic range is the ratio of the minimum detectable signal level (i.e., that measured to determine sensitivity) to the minimum signal required to saturate the system output. The minimum signal required to saturate the system can be determined with the same setup used to measure sensi-

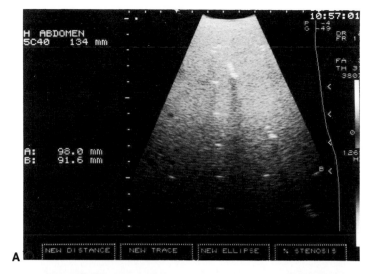

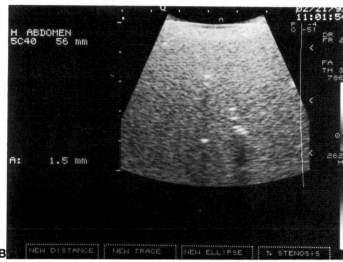

Fig. 13-8 (A) A large field-of-view image of RMI 413 phantom demonstrates registration accuracy and measurement calibration. Distance measurements are accurate within 2 percent both horizontally (1.6 mm in 90 mm) and vertically (2.0 mm in 100 mm). Depth of penetration is ~12 cm. **(B)** Magnified view of same phantom shows that this system has a negligible dead zone. Bright horizontal line is the layer of phantom. Resolution fibers, with nominal separations of 3 mm, 2 mm, 1 mm, and 0.5 mm, show an axial resolution on the order of 1 mm.

tivity, by increasing the excitation signal on the hydrophone to the point where the video signal is saturated. Typically, this test should be repeated for a receiver gain setting less than the maximum available, such as 6 dB below maximum.

Spatial Resolution

Spatial resolution is a three-dimensional quantity that can vary throughout the field of view. Quick estimates of spatial resolution in the image plane and in the elevation plane can be obtained using TM test objects.[1] These techniques, however, require that the system output control or gain control should be calibrated. If spatial resolution estimates are based on image brightness and the output and gains are not calibrated, the results often depend on the observer. Less subjective measures of spatial resolution can be obtained by mapping the pulse-echo response of the system using a small spherical reflector in a water tank. Using an example from optics, we can estimate the minimum resolvable separation between two point reflectors as the −6-dB pulse-echo lateral beamwidth (a variation on the Rayleigh criterion[12]). Near the radius of curvature, the beamwidth is approximately equal to $1.22\lambda z/D$, where λ is the wavelength of sound, z is the axial distance between the transducer and the field point, and D is the aperture size. For example, a 5-MHz transducer with an 80-mm focal length and a 30-mm aperture has a lateral resolution of approximately 1 mm near the focal length. If a hydrophone is used in place of the spherical reflector, the resulting beam profile represents properties of the beam during transmission only. Properties of the beam during reception may be estimated by recognizing that the pulse-echo lateral beam profile is given by the product of the transmitted and received lateral beam profiles. The pulse-echo axial beam profile is given by the convolution of the transmitted and received axial beam profiles.[5]

Spectral Response

The resonance frequency and pulse bandwidth of a transducer are important parameters that can be easily checked in an acoustics laboratory. Place a planar interface at the focus and align the transducer to receive the maximum echo signal amplitude. Digitally record the echo signal and calculate the signal spectrum. Half-amplitude (−6 dB) bandwidths of 50 to 60 percent are common for current transducer materials. For Gaussian-shaped pulses, the axial resolution, S_a, can be estimated from the −6-dB bandwidth, B, using $S_a \simeq 0.68/B$.

Transmit and Receive Apertures

Array aperture size can affect the system sensitivity and spatial resolution. A simple method for estimating the combined transmit–receive aperture involves the use of a small diameter wire (e.g., as a paper clip) acoustically coupled to the array.[13] As the array element below the wire is addressed for pulsing and receiving, an echo signal is produced by the wire, and the signal is displayed on the scanner monitor. By assuming that the receive aperture is larger than the transmit aperture, which is commonly true, the measurement yields the transmit aperture. The receive aperture can then be measured by placing a hydrophone in direct contact with the transducer surface. A CW signal is transmitted with the hydrophone at the resonance frequency of the array and received by the transducers. Aperture growth with image depth, transducer f-number, and receive apodization can all be shown with this technique. Transmit apodization can also be measured by listening with the hydrophone, instead of transmitting.

Photography

Ultrasound images recorded on photographic film are often the basis for diagnosis and therefore must be an accurate representation of the image viewed by the operator. A photograph of an image obtained from a TM phantom is a useful test of several parameters of the recording system. Scanning in a region where both horizontal and vertical rows of regularly spaced nylon wires are present provides an image to test for horizontal and vertical distortion in the recorded image. Most scanners provide a gray-scale bar near the edge of the image field to determine whether all shades of gray are being recorded on film.

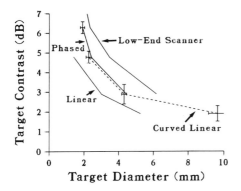

Fig. 13-9 Contrast-detail curves for four transducer technologies. Line indicates lowest target contrast observed for a given target diameter. Targets with properties that lie above a curve can be seen, so that lower curves represent transducers with greater low-contrast detectability.

Contrast-Detail Analysis

No scanner clearly outperforms competitors in its class at all the tasks so far discussed. In some cases, a summary measure of system performance at a specific but clinically essential task is desirable. Contrast-detail (CD) analysis is such a summary measure when it is important to detect low-contrast targets— as so often happens in general radiologic applications. CD analysis is a quick and easy alternative to standard receiver operating characteristic analyses. One application of CD analysis for evaluation of ultrasound imaging systems is shown in Figure 13-9. These preliminary data show that the low-contrast detectability of four transducer technologies can be quite different. These results, in conjunction with Equation 1, show how lesion detectability depends on specific elements of image quality.

FLOW MEASUREMENTS

The desire to quantitate flow velocities and volume flow rates places additional requirements on system performance. Flow volumes can be estimated when velocity profiles and vessel geometry are known. To estimate flow volumes accurately and to obtain high-precision Doppler spectra, it is necessary to determine the direction of flow within the vessel, not just the orientation of the vessel. These measurements are aided by visualizing the streamlines of flow, which requires high spatial and frequency resolution. Frequency resolution in Doppler measurements is analogous to gray-scale resolution in B-mode imaging. High spatial resolution provides estimates over small fluid volumes and more accurate estimates of vessel area; high-frequency resolution allows small increments in velocity to be detected for more accurate profiles. (A fundamental ambiguity restricts the frequency resolution possible for a given spatial resolution.[14]) Other parameters of interest are the sample volume size, location and angular orientation in a duplex Doppler system, and the sensitivity of the system for measuring low flow velocities in deep vessels.

Currently, there are no standards in the United States for acceptance testing of duplex Doppler or color-flow ultrasound equipment. Several methods have been reported for measuring important parameters. In addition to the test equipment already described, novel devices have been reported for some of the important tests, as described in the following sections.

Moving String Test Objects

Several authors have reported using moving strings as targets for flow test objects.[15-17] Some designs are commercially available (e.g., JJ&A Instruments, Redmond, Washington, and Nuclear Associates, Carle Place, New York). Moving string test objects are versatile devices that can be used to evaluate sample volume placement and profile, quadrature channel separation, flow angle indicator accuracy, and velocity calibration. Translating the transducer across the moving string provides a means to measure the beamwidth and sample volume. The string target also provides an easy method for testing registration of the sample volume location on the monitor. The ability to vary the string velocity allows measurement of the sensitivity and velocity resolution of the system, particularly for the condition where two strings are used to provide Doppler shifts from targets moving in different directions and at different velocities. Although this method is very useful, signal strengths of the moving target relative to the background medium (typically water) are much higher than that for blood and soft tissues. Also, the string does not provide the velocity variation normally seen in blood vessels, and the sample volume cannot be measured in all three directions.

Vibrating Point Target

A typical vibrating point target[18] is a 0.8-mm-diameter sphere mounted on a 0.01-mm-diameter wire and forced to oscillate axially at a frequency of approximately 500 Hz. This moving target provides a means of mapping the sample volume in three dimensions. It has been shown that the signal strength in the absence of the 0.8-mm sphere is insignificant. Thus, the echo signals originate primarily from the sphere. By moving the transducer in three dimensions above this target, the relative signal can be mapped to describe the sample volume.

Rotating Disk

Typically, a rotating disk target[19] can be used for measuring velocity accuracy over the range 1 to 1,000 cm/s. A slot cut in the perimeter of the disk provides a useful marker to indicate complete revolutions of the disk on the scanner monitor. With known rotational velocity and measurements from the monitor, calibration is easily verified. Modified rotational velocities are possible that simulate physiologic velocity patterns but are not necessary to verify calibration accuracy.

Flowing Fluid Test Objects

Several authors have reported using test objects that mimic blood flow in vessels.[20–22] Some designs are commercially available (e.g., RMI, Middleton, Wisconsin, and Echo Ultrasound, Lewistown, Pennsylvania). A fluid with acoustic properties similar to blood is pumped through plastic tubes to achieve constant flow or pulsatility similar to that in arteries and veins. These devices have been used to assess sample volume placement, quadrature channel separation, flow angle indicator accuracy, and velocity calibration using techniques similar to those for the moving string. A limitation of some of these implementations is that the flow profiles might not be stable along the length of the tubes. Transitions in tube diameters cause turbulence that can require long tube lengths to regain laminar flow, depending on volume flow rates.

Injected Signals

One alternative to test objects based on scanning moving objects is to inject signals into the imaging system. Thus, it is possible to use a pair of transducers, one to receive the scanner output and the other to transmit known signals, to test the accuracy of displayed frequency shifts, sample volume positioning, and system sensitivity.[23] The transducer pair and the probe from the system to be evaluated are coupled to a plastic block. The signal from the scanner is detected by the receiving transducer and mixed with the low-frequency signal produced by a local oscillator, thereby producing sum and difference frequencies and harmonics. These signals are sent back into the scanner through the transmitting transducer.

CONCLUSIONS

Engineering advances are beginning to reduce the need for routine monitoring of image quality in the clinical environment and to increase the need for effective acceptance testing procedures. Diagnostic performance is greatly affected by the choice of imaging probe and image processing for each patient examination. Therefore, to obtain the highest quality diagnosis, operators must understand the advantages and limitations of each system option. These can be discovered through knowledge of the technology and effective acceptance testing procedures.

REFERENCES

1. Standard Methods for Measuring Performance of Pulse-Echo Ultrasound Imaging Equipment. American Institute of Ultrasound in Medicine, Rockville, Maryland, 1991

2. Maslak SH: Computed sonography. p. 1. In Sanders RC, Hill MD (eds): Ultrasound Annual. Raven Press, New York, 1985

3. Wagner RF, Smith SW, Sandrik JM, Lopez H: Statistics of speckle in ultrasound B-scans. IEEE Trans Sonics Ultrason 30:156, 1983

4. Macovski A: Ultrasonic imaging using arrays. Proc IEEE 67:484, 1979

5. Wagner RF, Insana MF, Smith SW: Fundamental correlation lengths of coherent speckle in medical ultrasonic images. IEEE Trans Ultrason Ferroelect Freq Contr 35:34, 1988

6. Kremkau FW: Clinical benefit of higher acoustic output levels. Ultrasound Med Biol 15:69, 1989

7. Smith SW, Wagner RF, Sandrik JM, Lopez H: Low-contrast detectability and contrast/detail analysis in medical ultrasound. IEEE Trans Sonics Ultrason 30:164, 1983

8. Thijssen JM, Oosterveld BJ, Wagner RF: Gray level transforms and lesion detectability in echographic images. Ultrason Imaging 10: 171, 1988

9. Waag RC, Dalecki D, Smith WA: Estimate of wavefront distortion from measurements of scattering by model media and calf liver. J Acoust Soc Am 85:406, 1989

10. Nock L, Trahey GE, Smith SW: Phase aberration correction in medical ultrasound using speckle brightness as a quality factor. J Acoust Soc Am 85:1819, 1989

11. American Institute of Ultrasound in Medicine/National Electrical Manufacturers Association: Acoustic Output Measurement and Labeling Standard for Diagnostic Ultrasound Equipment. AIUM, Rockville, Maryland, 1989

12. Goodman JW: Introduction to Fourier Optics. McGraw-Hill, New York, 1968

13. Goldstein A, Ranney D, McLeary RD: Linear array test tool. J Ultrasound Med 8:385, 1989

14. Gill RW: Measurement of blood flow by ultrasound: accuracy and sources of error. Ultrasound Med Biol 11:625, 1985

15. Walker AR, Phillips DJ, Powers JE: Evaluating Doppler devices using a moving string test target. J Clin Ultrasound 10:25, 1982

16. Phillips DJ, Hossack J, Beach KW, Strandness DE: Testing ultrasonic pulsed Doppler instruments with a physiologic string phantom. J Ultrasound Med 9:429, 1990

17. Goldstein A: Performance tests of Doppler ultrasound equipment with a string phantom. J Ultrasound Med 10:125, 1991

18. Hoeks APG, Ruissen CJ, Hick P, Reneman RS: Methods to evaluate the sample volume of pulsed Doppler systems. Ultrasound Med Biol 10:427, 1984

19. Nelson TR, Pretorius DH: Device for the calibration of flow-velocity-measuring Doppler ultrasound equipment. J Ultrasound Med 9: 575, 1990

20. Smith HJ: Quantitative Doppler flowmetry. Acta Radiol Diagn 25:305, 1984

21. Boote EJ, Zagzebski JA: Performance tests of Doppler ultrasound equipment with a tissue and blood-mimicking phantom. J Ultrasound Med 7:137, 1988

22. Hoskins PR, Anderson T, McDicken WN: A computer controlled flow phantom for generation of physiological Doppler waveforms. Phys Med Biol 34:1709, 1989

23. Evans JA, Price R, Luhana F: A novel device for Doppler ultrasound equipment. Phys Med Biol 34:1701, 1989

Index

Page numbers followed by f indicate figures; those followed by t indicate tables.